HEADACHES
RELIEVED

For Mom and Dad, who suffered my headaches right along side me for so many decades. I love you.

HEADACHES RELIEVED

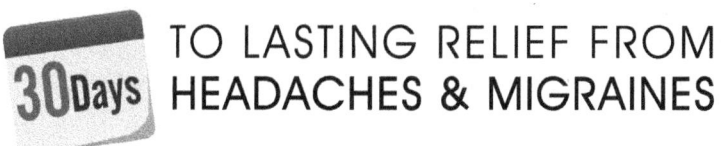
TO LASTING RELIEF FROM HEADACHES & MIGRAINES

DR. MARK WILEY

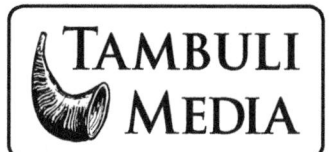

www.TambuliMedia.com
Spring House, PA USA

DISCLAIMER

The information in this book is provided for informational purposes only and is not a substitute for professional medical advice. The author and publisher make no legal claims, expressed or implied, and the material is not intended to replace the services of a physician.

The author, publisher and/or copyright holder assume no responsibility for the loss or damage caused, or allegedly caused, directly or indirectly by the use of information contained in this book. The author and publisher specifically disclaim any liability incurred from the use or application of the contents of this book.

All rights reserved. No part of this book may be reproduced or transmitted in any form by any means, electronic, mechanical, photocopying, recording or otherwise, without the prior written permission of the publisher.

Trademarked names appear throughout this book. Rather than place a trademark symbol next to every occurrence of a trademarked name, we use the names in an editorial fashion only and for the benefit of the trademark owner with no intention of infringement of the trademark.

Copyright © 2016 Mark V. Wiley. All rights reserved.
First published on March 20, 2017 by Tambuli Media

ISBN-10:0692865977
ISBN-13:978-0692865972
Library of Congress Control Number: 2016961537

Edited by Victoria Touati
Designed by Summer Bonne

PRAISE FOR DR. MARK WILEY'S
"Headache Relief Action Plan"

"Dr. Wiley's approach to headaches and migraines offers the most progressive focus available today."
—*Dr. Michael Maliszewski, Integrative Medicine Task Force*

"Dr. Wiley's personal suffering and tireless research into chronic headaches clearly shows that the only way to rid ourselves of them is through a self-directed and integrated mind-body approach. This book is a must. The results will amaze you!"
—*Dr. Robert Chu, Oasis Vitality Center*

"Dr. Wiley empowers readers to become active participants on a journey to health and wellness by presenting a detailed program, a GPS map and guide, including points of interest and alternate routes for reader to use and personalize their journey to becoming headache-free."
—*Dr. Christopher M. Viggiano, Chiropractic Physician*

"Dr. Mark Wiley has presented a truly extraordinary, experienced-based and scientifically designed approach to finding relief and long-term prevention of chronic headaches. His first-hand account, coupled with his 'Headache Relief Action Plan,' demonstrates how a complimentary and multi-dimensional approach can emerge as an innovative, comprehensive, and complete treatment program well within the reach of anyone actively seeking relief."
—*Dr. Juan Otero, Psychoanalyst and Certified Hypnotherapist*

"With the growing epidemic of headaches, this book is essential. Dr. Wiley's compelling story and self-directed program will give any headache sufferer the belief: 'If he can do it, so can I!'"
—*Dr. Brett Cardonick, Cardonick Chiropractic*

"Dr. Wiley is one of the clearest thinkers and writers in complimentary medicine today. I hope thousands of people will follow his plan and live the life they were born to enjoy."
—*Dr. Glenn P. Lobo, The Caring Osteopath*

"Dr. Mark Wiley is one of the most knowledgeable health and wellness experts I know. I'm certain you'll find this book to be an invaluable resource."
—*Jesse Cannone, CFT, CPRS, The Healthy Back Institute*

"Mark Wiley pulls no punches in empowering you to stop your headaches with a thorough integrative, natural, mind-body approach. I believe this program will do more for everyone than just cure headaches: It is a healing, healthy, preventative lifestyle for us all! Read it. Do it. And Enjoy life again."
—*Gary D. Sandman, Individual Health Solutions*

"Combining the latest Western medical research with proven Eastern medical techniques, Dr. Wiley presents a fully integrated approach to eliminating headaches forever. If you suffer from this kind of pain, your path to recovery begins with this book."
—*Brian Saint-Paul, Editor, CRISIS Magazine*

"In my years of clinical Chinese medicine practice, I have found Dr. Wiley's self-help headache program to be the best in terms of headache treatment."
—*Alan Orr, LAc, The Chinese Medicine Academy*

"Not only is Headaches Relieved well researched, it is a well-rounded example of how to integrate healthy lifestyle modifications to enhance your overall quality of life. As a future physician, I am pleased that this book is available as a resource for those suffering from chronic headache pain."
—*Vico M. Viggiano, Rowan University School of Osteopathic Medicine*

This book is for YOU

– the headache sufferer –

who is tired of letting

pain control your life.

In these pages,

you will find the

keys to lasting relief.

A WORD OF CAUTION

Although the "Headache Relief Action Plan" presented in this book is a powerful healing system, there are times when headache pain requires immediate medical attention. According to the National Institute of Neurological Disorders and Stroke (NINDS), you should seek prompt medical care if you experience any of the following...

- ✓ An abrupt, severe headache or a sudden headache associated with a stiff neck
- ✓ A headache associated with fever or convulsions or accompanied by confusion or loss of consciousness
- ✓ A headache following a blow to the head or associated with pain in the eye or ear.
- ✓ Persistent headache in a person who was previously headache-free
- ✓ Recurring headaches in children

TABLE OF CONTENTS

Foreword by Dr. Michael Maliszewski i

Foreword by Dr. Christopher M. Viggiano iv

A Personal Message from Dr. Mark Wiley 1

Introduction: A Headache-free Life is Your Birthright! 7

PART 1: THE MANY MYTHS, TYPES AND TRIGGERS OF HEADACHES AND MIGRAINES

Chapter 1: The Eight Biggest Headache Myths 17

Chapter 2: Headache Types and Triggers 29

Chapter 3: How Mainstream Medicine Can Make Headaches Worse 45

Chapter 4: The 15 Biggest Headache Mistakes People Make .. 55

Chapter 5: How Food Impacts Headache and Migraine 75

Chapter 6: How Stress and Emotions Affect Headaches 89

Chapter 7: The Three Hidden Imbalances That Cause Headaches 97

PART 2: NATURAL SOLUTIONS YOUR DOCTOR DOESN'T KNOW

Chapter 8: Avoiding the Pitfall of Wrong Treatment 109

Chapter 9: The Headache Prevention Diet 117

Chapter 10: Supplements for Headache Relief and Prevention 135

Chapter 11: Stress Reduction and Meditation for Headache Relief.. 151

Chapter 12: Breathing Exercises for Headache Relief.......... 161

Chapter 13: Sleep Your Way to Headache Relief................. 169

Chapter 14: Releasing the Pain Body for Headache Relief.. 181

Chapter 15: Stretching and Bodywork for Headache Relief 195

Chapter 16: Ancient Exercises for Headache Relief.............211

Chapter 17: Energy Medicine for Headache Relief..............229

Chapter 18: Unusual Interventions for Headache Relief......245

Chapter 19: Pain Relief Interventions for Specific Headache Locations..253

PART 3: THE 30-DAY HEADACHE RELIEF ACTION PLAN

Chapter 20: Introduction to the Headache Relief Action Plan..267

Chapter 21: A Positive Attitude Supports a Successful Program 271

Chapter 22: Setting SMART Wellness Goals for Success......277

Chapter 23: Program Strategies, Objectives and Metrics 283

Chapter 24: Getting Started: The First Three Days................305

Chapter 25: Step-by-Step: The 30-Day Headache Relief Action Plan 311

Afterword..321

References...323

About Dr. Mark Wiley 330

FOREWORD BY
DR. MICHAEL MALISZEWSKI

Headache disorders constitute one of the most debilitating health problems in the world today. More than 45 million people in the United States have chronic headaches. Out of this amount, some 11 million have severe headaches that lead to some type of disability. The World Health Organization (WHO) has estimated that nearly half of the adult population has experienced headache pain at least once in the past year. Despite advances in medical treatment, the growing body of research and interventions in medical and scientific literature, and the addition of articles on the topic gaining popularity on the Internet, significant changes leading to reduction in headache incidence have remained elusive to date.

I am pleased to write a foreword to Dr. Mark Wiley's new book, *Headaches Relieved*. I have known Mark for over 20 years. We have shared parallel paths of investigation, and sought out the most effective techniques, procedures, programs, and practitioners professing to have the best and most comprehensive approach to pain management and control, that result in reduction of severe conditions and symptoms of headache pain. I believe Mark's approach to pain management is "cutting edge," and offers the most progressive focus available today as compared to other strategies currently present in the healthcare field.

My professional background is germane to writing this foreword. Initially trained as a clinical psychologist at the University of Chicago, I later went on to develop the world's largest, single-site behavioral medicine program at the Diamond Headache Clinic in Chicago—a setting which treats some 20,000 patients internationally and annually for headache pain and related disorders. Using an approach known as Accelerated Behavioral Medicine (ABM), the design of the ABM program was to assess headache pain conditions and offer the most rapid strategies to reduce pain through non-pharmacological, psychological and psychophysical interventions with a maximum time being less than three hours to effectively convey and complete the holistic treatment protocol. This approach contrasts greatly with other pain treatment programs available that involve anywhere from two weeks to several months of training to participate in and gain results. Eight years later, I became associated with the psychology/psychiatry department at Massachusetts General Hospital (MGH)/Harvard Medical School, and served as a consultant at that setting for 20 years. Currently, I conduct private practice consultation and I am a member of the Integrative Medicine Task Force at Spaulding Hospital in Boston, another Harvard-based hospital affiliated with MGH. In addition, I have received grants to travel and conduct field research on indigenous healing traditions throughout nearly a dozen Asian countries, as well as for investigating pain programs throughout the USA and Europe.

Sharing a similar thirst for knowledge and discovery, Mark Wiley and I became familiar with one another's work, research, and writings, and recognized how truly limited was the background and method other programs and practitioners were offering pain relief solutions to their clients. Our parallel approaches entailed what might be termed an "evidence-based practice" to testing the most viable and successful strategies to pain control within ourselves and with our clients.

I cannot emphasize enough the importance of the "Headache Relief Action Plan" approach Dr. Wiley presents in this book. This is not simply a compendium of techniques currently popular in the literature or found in online searches. Nor is it an advertisement to argue the superiority of one method, approach or program over another. It goes much deeper. A basic tenet is that a combination of various therapies and approaches offer the best chance for improvement. But even more relevant, it stresses the importance of self-administration of pain-relieving techniques where the pain sufferer takes control of his or her conditions(s) directly and initiates and pursues an individualized, self-design module rather than relying exclusively on some external program or practitioner to alleviate the pain for them. A psychologist might describe it as a shift in "locus of control" from external agent and back to the person themselves. This is unique among the most popular programs today that offer highly publicized approaches and outcomes in the media, but are also quite expensive in terms of costs (financial as well as time invested).

Headaches Relieved is a welcome breath of fresh air for acute and chronic headache and migraine sufferers who either need a little help or are at their wit's end with unsuccessful headache pain management. All it takes is the motivated individual who wants to lead a healthy and pain-free lifestyle with minimal inconveniences and seeks to initiate a positive opportunity for further growth and freedom from pain.

Michael Maliszewski, PhD
Integrative Medicine Taskforce

FOREWORD BY DR. CHRISTOPHER M. VIGGIANO

It is with great honor and poignancy I endorse my fellow colleague, Dr. Mark Wiley, as a practitioner of the medicinal, meditational, and martial art disciplines. Dr. Wiley has dedicated his unwavering passion as a physician and educator to help guide his patients and students through turbulent waters towards the hidden gems of eternal, inherent wisdom, good health and pain-free living.

In *Headaches Relieved*, Dr. Wiley sheds light on the inefficiency of pills, powders & potions to treat headaches, and walks readers through a new approach to treating the myriad of headache-related disorders and diseases, as well as identifying their proper diagnosis and treatments.

Dr. Wiley explains how stress, food, water, and air can contribute or detract from one's health and make one susceptible to chronic headaches and migraines. Having also suffered from severe, debilitating headaches since childhood, Dr. Wiley shares his knowledge and self-healing methods for treating headaches and migraines, which he acquired through his education, travels, research, and personal experience. By identifying the underlying causes of headaches, one can significantly reduce the frequency and severity of chronic headaches and migraines.

From his extensive research and development, Dr. Wiley empowers readers to become active participants on a journey to health and wellness by presenting a detailed outline called the "Headache Relief Action Plan," which contains a map and guide (a GPS, if you will), including points of interest and alternate routes for reader to use and personalize on their journey to becoming headache-free.

In conclusion, this valuable book is for all seekers of truth who are ready and willing to adopt and adapt transformational changes into their personal lifestyle that will activate the innate, inborn rejuvenating healing life-force of mind-body-spirit synergy.

As inspired patients, you need only to supply the will, and Dr. Mark Wiley will provide a way.

Dr. Christopher M. Viggiano
Chiropractic Physician & Health Care Consultant
Martial Arts Researcher, Developer & Educator
Fellow Headache Sufferer

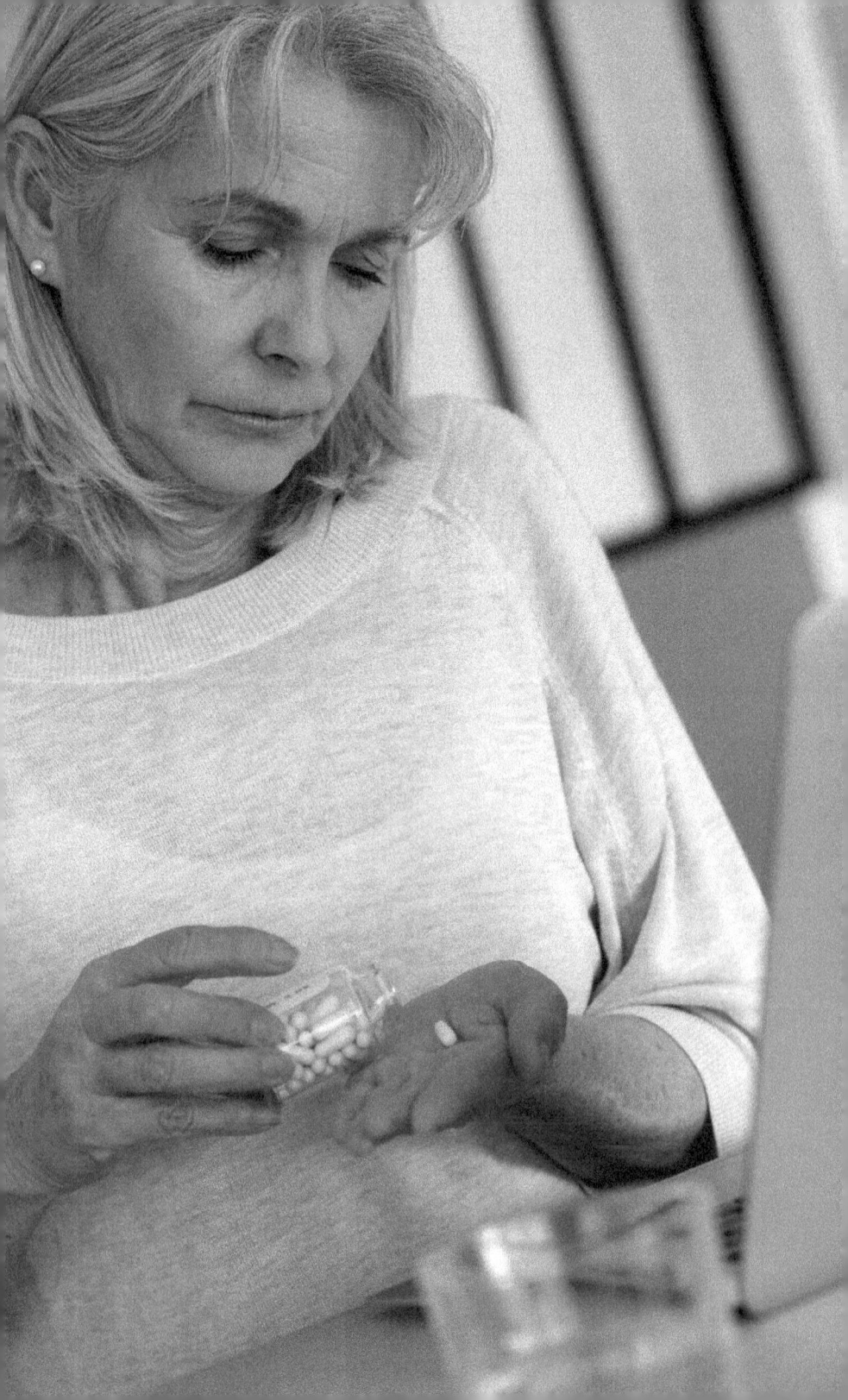

A PERSONAL MESSAGE FROM DR. MARK WILEY

Headaches are one of the most common disorders known to man, and the human race has been suffering from them since the beginning of time. Everything has been done to try to cure them: from drilling of the skull and bloodletting to prescription drug therapy and surgery. Yet, the challenge to prevent headaches, to find a cure and to bring relief is ever present in every country around the world.

The basic problem headache sufferers face is the complexity of their condition. Not all headaches are the same; not everyone experiences headaches and their symptoms the same way, and the same trigger does not always cause the same type of headache. What's more, headaches encompass physical, physiological and emotional dimensions. In short, they are complex structures that need a comprehensive approach to achieve their banishment.

Hello, I'm Dr. Mark Wiley and I want to ask you something: Do you get headaches? How often and how bad are they? Do they control your life? Do you feel at times like giving up and not going on?

The reason I ask is because that's how I felt every day for over three decades. But, during this time, I was also deeply involved in martial arts and traditional spiritual practices so I kept telling myself, "I'm the King of Pain. I can take this. I can wait it out and defeat it."

What were my migraines like? Life shattering and soul destroying. For instance, one fall day, as I walked along Philadelphia's Schuylkill River, positive thoughts of the future filled my mind. Life was good. Twenty seconds later, during the onset of a migraine, I wanted to die.

It struck from behind like a truck slamming into a wall. Pain seared through my head as effortlessly as a chainsaw glides through balsawood. My head felt like it was being crushed from the outside and pushed apart from the inside at the same time. At the same time, it was like someone was jamming a screwdriver into my right eye, and a rock was being wedged under the base of my skull. Shivers, cold sweats and shaky knees forced me to drop in pain, gasping for air.

To deaden the pain, I began scraping my forehead across the ground and then along the cool stone wall. Lunch came back up on me as violently as a dam suddenly broken by the force of a raging flood. Deep, dark spots and burning tears obstructed my vision as I begged for death. But I was intimate with this pain, and knew very well that neither death nor God would come to my rescue.

And yet, this was only an average attack; not even close to being one of the worst. It was just another in the life-long series of daily migraine, and cluster, tension, toxic and rebound headaches I had experienced for nearly three decades. My migraines persisted EVERY DAY, despite taking an average of 14 capsules of various medications a day and having seen and been treated by some of the best-trained physicians of Western medicine.

The constant, uncontrollable suffering was destroying me. I couldn't exercise on a regular basis because of severe headaches caused by jumping, running and lifting. This was particularly demoralizing as I was a professional martial artist. During college, as a result of being bed-ridden, I had to do extracurricular work to make up for missed classes and exams. I knew if the headaches kept recurring on this schedule for much longer I would, in the immortal words of Ed Grimly, "Go mental!"

You see, I began life 2-½ months premature, weighing in at only 1 pound, 9 ounces. My first four months were spent in the hospital. I had below average bone development, experienced breathing difficulties, and suffered infantile spasms, which are now believed to have been deep seizures. Doctors now think all this resulted in the chronic musculoskeletal pain and mixed headaches that dogged me since childhood (or perhaps birth).

My parents selflessly spent a tremendous amount of time and money trying to cure these pains the Western way, but to no avail. By the time I was 13, I was experiencing "rebound" headaches—additional headaches caused by the body's reaction to the combination and large volume of prescription and over-the-counter medications in my system. At different times, I was prescribed beta blockers, and calcium channel blocker drugs. At one point, I was taking a combination of two Midrin, two Fioricet and two Excedrin at one swallow—several times a day! This powerful migraine treatment didn't always relieve the pain, nor did it keep my headaches from recurring. When the prescription capsules were unable to do their job, and my headache pain was so severe and debilitating, I would be taken to the emergency room where both Demurral and Samaritan were administered intravenously along with Zofran for nausea and vomiting. Even with this mixture, it would often take an additional four hours for the pain to dissipate. In short, while Western methods did treat the symptoms of the headache (i.e., pain, aura, cold sweats, nausea), they did my headache pain no lasting good and caused short-term harm to my body.

In 1982, when I was 13, my father introduced me to his chiropractor, and this visit began my journey into alternative health and wellness. I spent the better part of the 1990s traveling around the world to meet with traditional healers in the United States, Japan, Taiwan, Malaysia, Singapore, Hong Kong, and the Philippines. I sought out those rumored to be Eastern geniuses of so-called "alternative" and "holistic" medicine, whose patients reached their waiting rooms by climbing mountains or hacking through jungles. Acupuncturists in Japan, Qigong masters in Taiwan, bone setters in Malaysia, faith healers in the Philippines... I've been there, done that.

To my dismay, I found that while their methods of diagnosis and treatment are diametrically opposed to, and far less toxic than the Western model, their treatments actually offered no greater, long-term relief from my chronic headaches.

Then it happened: One morning I just woke up and decided I had had enough. I decided to take my health and well-being into my own hands, rather than expecting someone else to take care of them for me. I read every book and journal study I could find on headache etiology and treatment. I met with leading experts in Western pain management and Eastern alternative therapies to discuss the topic and my condition and observations. It wasn't until I stepped back from the forest that I saw the trees, each one of them individually, for the first time. It was then that I began to really understand the variety of factors causing my headaches, and the answer to eliminating the so-called "triggers" from my life, and, by extension, the headaches themselves.

What is the bottom line in my story?

After more than 30 years of skull-melting, eye-blinding headache pain, I finally reached the top of the mountain, put all the wisdom together—conventional and unconventional—and I am here to tell you, I killed the monsters forever. And now I want to tell you how you can kill them, too, and get on with a life worth living.

To come to the point where you are psychologically ready to stop playing the role of victim to the headache and servant to the physician/healer takes great courage and discipline. I am confident you have what it takes to outwit your headaches and take back control of your life. So do it. I encourage you to do it now, without another moment's delay. I promise your life will change in innumerable ways with the coming of lasting pain relief. Do it now, because no one except you gives a damn about the quality of *your* life. This book will show you the way. All you have to do is make and keep a personal promise and commitment to yourself that you will see The Headache Relief Action Plan through to the end.

I was able to do it. And I know you can do it, too.

I believe in you!

Dr. Mark Wiley

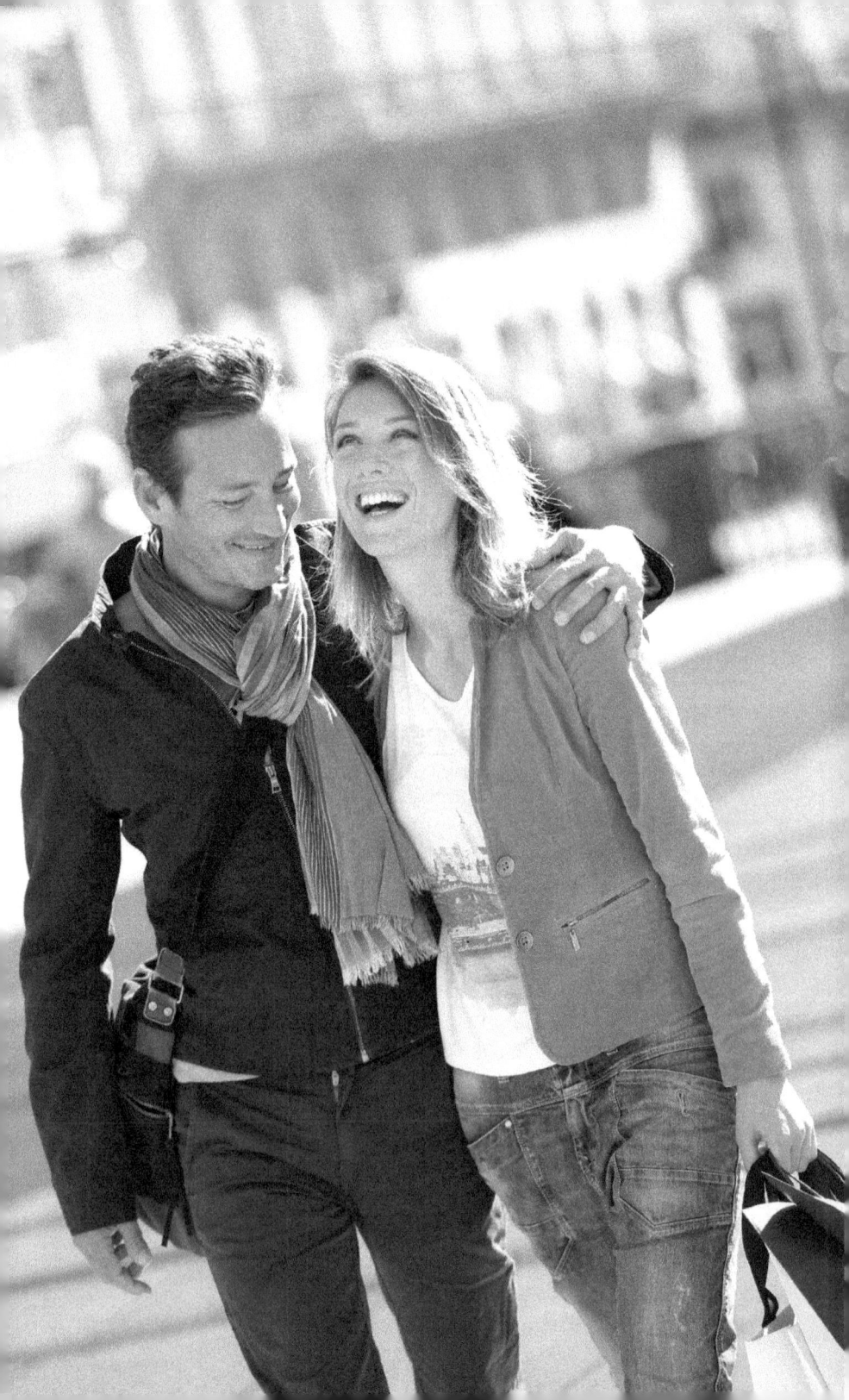

INTRODUCTION

A HEADACHE-FREE LIFE IS YOUR BIRTHRIGHT!

A joyous, headache-free life is your birthright and within the pages of this book I am going to show you how to reclaim that right. You see, I've spent over three decades researching and mastering natural wellness practices around the world. I've taken those techniques and pioneered a powerful integrated mind-body approach to well-being and pain-free living. It's a self-directed, do-it-yourself (DIY) kind of approach. And, it is based on this fundamental truth:

> *You don't have to live in pain.*
> *You don't have to suffer a chronic health condition.*
> *The migraines and headaches you "deal with" every day*
> *do not need to be permanent fixtures in your life.*
> *I will tell you why and show you how to overcome them.*

I know you wish it were true… and I am here to tell you, it is!

Yet, from early on, you are taught to "manage" and "mask" the symptoms of and "live with" your poor health conditions. This is perverse. It goes against our homeostatic (self-balancing) nature. What's more, despite lackluster results, too many people keep following the practices of a healthcare system that simply has not delivered on its promises.

Are we doing this because we don't realize it's not working? Surely, our chronic daily pain and suffering is the indication it's not working.

Chronic headaches and migraines are a massive problem that destroys lives. A quick look at statistics presented by the World Health Organization (WHO), tells a terrible tale[1]:

- Headache disorders are among the most common disorders of the nervous system.
- It has been estimated that almost half of the adult population have had a headache at least once within the last year.
- Between 50% and 75% of adults all over the world had a headache within the preceding year.
- In the United States, over 15% of all adults complain about severe headaches or migraines.
- Episodic tension headaches, ones that occur fewer than 15 days per month, are reported by more than 70% of some populations.
- Headache disorders, characterized by recurrent headaches, are associated with personal and societal burdens of pain, disability, damaged quality of life, and financial cost.
- Worldwide, a minority of people with headache disorders are diagnosed appropriately by healthcare providers.
- Headaches have been underestimated, under-recognized and under-treated throughout the world.

Chronic headaches produce insufferable pain and suffering.

Simply put, mainstream medicine fails to eradicate our everyday pains, illnesses and diseases. It fails because it offers only a passive and *reactionary* model of treating patients and disease, and, thus unable to prevent you from experiencing chronic health conditions such as heart disease, diabetes, hypertension, obesity, stress, anxiety, depression, headaches and migraines, back pain, tendonitis and hundreds of other illnesses.

And this model will always fall short because it uses *disease* as its basis of finding *health*. The way this works is you see your primary care physician when you are ill; the doctor diagnoses your illness, labels the disease and then prescribes a protocol for treating the disease or symptoms. Your personal health issues are "managed" by prescription medication, various therapies and surgery. Natural treatment can also fall into this category, if the approach is relief of symptoms and not correction of the underlying (root) causes. While treating symptoms of pain and inflammation are necessary for immediate relief, it must be done as an intermediary step while implementing a truly corrective approach, such as the one presented in this book. After all, any model based simply on symptomatic relief (whether modern or traditional) can never hope to resolve your daily wellness problems.

As a person suffering with headaches and migraines, the important thing is to see and know the solution to your daily suffering is grounded in a five-part process I call the "Headache Relief Action Plan." This plan consists of the following parts:

The "Headache Relief Action Plan"

Part 1: Educate yourself about the myths, triggers and solutions of headaches

Part 2: Reduce the level of pain and symptoms you experience with headaches

Part 3: Halt and significantly reduce the frequency and duration of your headaches

Part 4: Prevent the headaches from being triggered to improve your quality of life

Part 5: Reestablish balance in the body to change its interior environment that allows headaches to manifest

These five parts can be achieved. In fact, for the best and fastest results, you should work toward them at the same time. With the exception of educating yourself on what to do and how to do it, one part does not come before the other. I have written this book with the express purpose of delivering all the information you need to satisfy all five parts of the headache equation in one place.

When it comes to headache relief and prevention, I am sure you have spoken to many specialists. You may be wondering why you should you believe in what I say. Well, for starters, I know how you feel. Like you, I went from doctor to doctor, desperately hoping for relief, but no one could help me. Every day was a soul-destroying battle with neck and shoulder pain, mid-back pain, hip pain and head pain. Pain, pain, pain.

Unlike some chronic pain sufferers, I was fortunate enough to have familial support growing up. Both of my parents were healthcare professionals: my father was an osteopathic physician and my mother was a psychologist. Unfortunately, even with their love, direction and referral to experts in various specialties, the suffering was constant, unbearable and unrelenting. I was forever putting myself in front of medical doctors, osteopaths, naturopaths, chiropractors, physical therapists, psychologists, allergists, body workers, hypnotists and dietitians. No treatment or surgery had lasting results.

I became proactive in college. In addition to studying medical anthropology, I was in close contact with dozens of mind-body health practitioners around the country. I became a research assistant at Harvard Medical School, and worked on how to combine various mind-body methods for pain relief, as well as researching the creation and use of specific martial art drills to create altered states of consciousness. Yet, despite all this, the net results were underwhelming. I was finally forced to face the fact that conventional Western medicine and many of the so-called "complementary medicines" were unable to heal me. So I became the Marco Polo of pain.

As I mentioned in the previous section, I travelled the world in search of cures for pain and suffering, often these cures had strange-sounding names: Reiki and Zen meditation in Japan, Qigong and Tuina in Taiwan, acupuncture and traditional herbs in Singapore, faith healing and bone-setting in the Philippines, medicine men and kundalini healers in Malaysia. I tried them all, and like Western medicine, there was some short-term relief, but my headaches and migraines always returned. Always. Then one day, I had enough and decided to make a final desperate change in my life's direction.

What did I do?

I started by going back to school to acquire knowledge in anatomy and physiology in order to better understand and assimilate the methods of the great healing traditions. I earned a Master's Degree in Health Care Management and doctorates in Acupuncture and Oriental Medicine (OMD) and Alternative Medicine (PhD). After 15 years of treating patients, teaching worldwide and writing books and hundreds of articles, I developed a proactive, self-directed, self-cure model of optimal health and pain-free living. The invaluable information found in this book is derived from the principles of that method. The solutions for each specific disease or condition – like headaches and migraines – is set into the plan template, for specificity.

The "Headache Relief Action Plan" entails some key lifestyle changes. These are necessary when it comes to defeating the debilitating triggers and symptoms of acute and chronic headaches and migraines. While lifestyle changes are the only way to correct imbalances, and *remain in an optimal state of health,* they are not always difficult. Sure, some of these changes may be more difficult than others for some people to implement and adopt, depending on their habits. But, some of the suggested changes are very simple and even fun to take up.

With this in mind, *Headaches Relieved* is divided into three parts. Each part should be read consecutively in the order it's presented for best results. Please do not skip ahead. Read everything first, keeping in mind that the first part of the five-part program is "educating yourself" on the true cause, triggers and myths about headaches and migraines.

Part 1: The Many Causes, Triggers and Myths of Headaches aims to educate you on the how's, why's and what's of headaches and migraines in easily understood language with no jargon and more explanation. By understanding the headache and migraine situation from many perspectives (not just medical, but holistic and alternative, too), you will see the condition for what it really is. This section lays out the *obvious* and *hidden causes* of headaches and migraines and the things that make it worse – many of which you have direct control over through aligning your choices with a headache-free lifestyle.

Part 2: Natural Solutions Your Doctor Doesn't Know provides an overview of the most powerful and accessible treatment options for headache and migraine. It discusses both Eastern and Western methods from bodywork to energy medicine to pain creams, diet and supplementation. It offers a broad view on the many options available to you for relief, some of which you may not have been aware of. It gives insights into each option so you can find one or several that work best for you.

Part 3: The 30-Day Headache Relief Action Plan is set into three "30-Day Action Plans" that pull all this information together for you. It provides the "how to do it" approach using a series of steps and an action plan you can implement over a brief period to achieve the five-part solution mentioned above. Its only aim is to provide you with a map that leads to headache relief and prevention, ultimately creating a better quality of life for you.

I would like to stress how important it is to have a mentor when dealing with health and wellness. It is difficult to do on your own, even with the hundreds of self-help articles at your fingertips on the Internet. Sure, a day spent surfing the Net could turn up hundreds of separate articles that discuss some of the things found in this book. But, would that be enough? I don't think so. Without a context in which to understand and place the information, how can you hope to implement it in an appropriate and significant way? I have the education and personal chronic headache experience necessary to assimilate the individual parts of the headache puzzle and then present to you the parts as a cohesive whole. So let me be your mentor, and let this book provide you with the proper context in which to understand headaches, their symptoms and the methods available to overcome their debilitating effects on your life.

In the pages of this book, I show you how to determine the underlying – and sometimes hidden – causes (or triggers) of your headaches and migraines. These are actually obvious root causes and contributors that are only "hidden" because you have not (yet) been taught to look for and identify them. I'll show you how to do this and then how to use that knowledge to reduce your headache triggers and symptoms, typically within 30 to 90 days. The information and plan is comprehensive, easy-to-understand and set out in a way that you can follow. And don't worry: what you'll discover in the following pages will pass your "common sense" test with flying colors. As you read, you'll find yourself nodding along and telling yourself, "Yes, this makes sense." The information and program outlined in this book works, so let's get started on overcoming your headaches and migraines so you, too, can live a headache-free life.

PART 1

THE MANY MYTHS, TYPES AND TRIGGERS OF HEADACHES AND MIGRAINES

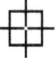

Acupuncture Cluster

Diet Tension-type

Stress **?** Female

Herbs

Myths ———△——— Facts

Drugs

Headache

Male

Migraine

CHAPTER 1

THE EIGHT BIGGEST HEADACHE MYTHS

To be successful at any endeavor, you must first understand the whole of that undertaking. When it comes to making a plan that works and sticking to it, you must also avoid the pitfalls. When it comes to a subject as complex as headaches and migraines, one must have clarity, and be able to separate myth from fact.

For you to be successful in implementing the "Headache Relief Action Plan," there must be a clear understanding of all the components involved in headache and migraine triggers, relief and prevention. This begins with clearing up the myths and setting forth the facts of the situation, and this is the intent of this chapter.

The line between fact and fiction is often thin. People form beliefs on what they think sounds *reasonable* and their knowledge of a specific topic, whether they gain that information from a friend, doctor, read it in a magazine or online or learn about it on the news. Myths in healthcare take shape (and indeed take on a life of their own) when a sound bite or piece of information (known today as a meme) is spread and made public as fact before the person or company releasing the information has the necessary *context* in which to consider the so-called facts. Without a context in which to understand something, any piece of content (information) is meaningless.

When it comes to complex conditions such as headaches and migraines, the pain and symptoms can wreak havoc on a life. As a person suffering from headaches, you already know how difficult it can be to maintain your quality of life, daily routines, and a cheery disposition and positive outlook. This is especially true during times of extreme pain and immobility. Please know and believe me when I say, "Severe pain, immobility and negative outlook do not have to be the center of your life." This book aims to help you believe and learn how to live pain free.

In the following pages, I briefly outline eight of the most common myths surrounding headaches and migraines. Please take your time as you read this chapter and consider each myth. For those myths you believe, be open to understanding the myths and then to believing the facts.

It is my sincere hope that by understanding these basic yet simple facts, you will find a more positive view of your condition, and, as a result, be more inclined to follow the therapeutic solutions found in later chapters. After all, a firm belief based in fact goes a long way toward beginning and maintaining a wellness program, especially when one is facing daily pain and physical and emotional debilitation. Let's take a look at those myths.

MYTH #1
All Headaches Are the Same

One of the most pervasive myths of all is the notion there is only one type of headache and migraine and it just happens to have different symptoms for different people. Some experience them as sinus pressure, some beginning with tension in the neck, but, regardless of how they begin they are all the same condition.

It is easy to see how people might think headaches are a single condition. After all, many headache types share common triggers, and they all have pain in the head as their main symptom. But the fact is, there are over 30 different types of headaches and migraines, which are divided into primary and secondary types. Everyone gets headaches for different reasons and the same reason can trigger different headaches in different people. So just because you know someone who may also have chronic headaches doesn't meant that what worked or failed for them will work or fail for you as well.

Just having basic clarity on this myth alone should provide you with some anxiety relief about the future potential of your headache-free life goal. Moreover, because a headache is not a disease but a symptom of a problem, and those problems are varied and not all applicable to your situation, the future can become clearer as you read this book.

Simply knowing headaches are not a single disease, but various head-pain-related symptoms caused by imbalances within the body that can be managed and corrected with natural, non-invasive approaches should provide you with enough hope for change that you find almost immediate improvement in your daily outlook.

MYTH #2
Migraines Are Just Bad Headaches

Continuing our discussion regarding Myth #1, there are 30 different kinds of headaches. Migraines are among the worst and certainly take a toll. For many, just hearing the diagnosis "migraine" or assuming it is enough to cause emotional stress, worry and depression about one's future.

The fact is that headaches and migraines are different things. Migraine is a narrowly specific type of headache based in temporary neurological dysfunction. Most headaches do not fall into this category or share the same symptoms of aura, nausea, sweating, and prolonged pain for days as migraines.

Migraines are relatively rare when compared to tension type headaches, which are due to muscle contraction around the shoulders and neck and cause referred pain to the head. Putting to bed the myth that migraines are the same as bad headaches should provide relief in your outlook and expectations.

MYTH #3
Only Women Get Migraines

While it is true that more women than men get migraines, they are not limited to women. The fact is that anyone can experience a migraine, including children. The statistics of the World Health Organization (WHO) show that migraine strike 18% of women, 8% of men, and 10% of children. It is a myth to believe that only women get migraines; however, they are serious and need be treated so keep an open mind and read on to see how to distinguish whether you are experiencing migraines or another kind of headache. The good news is the "Headache Relief Acton Plan" address all types of headaches.

MYTH #4
Headaches Are a Normal Part of Life

It is easy to see how this myth (and similar ones relating to health) took hold. A simple look at the people around you, the commercials on television and the shelves in pharmacies seems to reinforce the idea that "everyone" gets headaches. While this may be an accurate assessment, it is not a "truth" that headaches are a normal or natural part of life.

To begin correcting this myth, it is important to know that headaches are symptoms and, therefore, have nothing to do with any "normal" part of life. Most headaches are simply the result of a combination of poor lifestyle choices. That is to say, they are triggered by factors like diet, level of exercise, sleep patterns, stress levels, posture, use of chemical cleaners in the home, how often we drink alcohol, and many other things. By changing your lifestyle choices, and altering your activities in daily life, you can reduce the triggers and stop the headache cycles.

MYTH #5
If You Have Headaches or a Migraine, You Should Not Exercise

This myth is most believed by those suffering with headaches because, well, it hurts a lot to exercise when you have a headache. Also, when you have chronic migraines, the days between episodes are filled with rest to recuperate and regain your energy. So, exercise is the last thing people with headaches think about.

While it is true that certain exercises, such as jumping and running, should be avoided, to prevent certain types and conditions of headaches and migraines, this is not a blanket statement to stop all forms of exercise.

The first step is to begin exercising slowly, lightly, and within limits so as not to worsen or aggravate headache or migraine conditions. Exercises like walking, yoga, Tai chi, Qigong, and even Pilates are good for those who get headaches. The more you can do, beginning slowly at first and more over time, the more you can increase your vitality and reduce certain headache and migraine triggers.

MYTH #6
The Environment Has No Effect on Headaches and Migraines

The very opposite of this myth is true and people who experience chronic headaches can usually attribute them to a time and place. In my own personal experience, I would get headaches in some department stores but not in others; when getting off airplanes; and right before or after a rain storm or on extremely humid days or in damp basements. My other headache triggers included every time I was in a room cleaned with Pine-Sol or Pledge, and spending time in overcrowded, developing tropical cities in Southeast Asia.

All of my headache trigger examples had an environmental issue in play that includes air quality (i.e., pressure, humidity, pollution), the ratio of negative to positive ions in the atmosphere, the quantity of toxic chemicals used to clean clothing or surfaces you normally come into contact with, the relative stuffiness and heat of a room, and the type of lighting used to illuminate a work, shopping or living space.

Flickering fluorescent lights, perfumes, dust, pollution, humidity and too many positive ions in the air are all potential migraine triggers. Many migraineurs complain they feel either better or worse around a thunderstorm. This happens for several reasons, two of which include changing humidity levels (for better or worse, depending on the temperature), which affects headaches, and the increased release of negative ions after a rainfall. The higher the concentration of positive ions and levels of relative humidity, the greater the chances of a migraine being triggered.

A study published in the journal *Neurology*[1], looked at over 7,000 patients who visited the emergency department (ED) of hospitals for severe headaches. In this study, they also examined the occurrence of higher temperatures and lower barometric pressures in the environment of each participant. The researchers compared levels of temperature, barometric pressure, humidity, fine particulate matter, black carbon, and nitrogen and sulfur dioxides during the three 24-hour periods preceding the emergency department (ED) visit for each headache patient. They found a 7.5% higher risk of severe headache reported for each temperature increase of 9 degrees Fahrenheit, and, to a lesser but still evident degree, a spike with lower barometric pressure 48 to 72 hours prior to patients' ED visits.

While the above study did not find a direct correlation with air pollution, a meta-analysis[2] looked at the impact of air pollution on migraines and headaches and concluded: "Available evidence supports the idea of a positive association between levels of some outdoor air pollutants and increased severity, frequency or medical consultation rates for headache and migraine. These effects occur across the spectrum of headache severity, ranging from increased frequency or duration of headaches that do not prompt medical consultation to an increase in the occurrence of more severe headaches that result in ED visits and even hospitalization. This suggests that pollutants are environmental irritants that right-shift the severity curve in the headache-susceptible population."

MYTH #7
There's No Cure for Headaches and Migraines

This myth is harmful and holds people hostage to the false idea they have to live in pain. It's total crap so please do not give it power over you. Yet this huge myth is widely believed. Why? Because many headache and migraine sufferers *do* live in pain, with chronic headaches and migraine episodes. They are suffering greatly, yet needlessly. Why? Because they don't know all of the parts of the headache and migraine puzzle. Knowing them instills knowledge and knowledge provides the impetus and power for change.

By engaging in mind-body exercises to reduce stress, eating an anti-inflammatory diet, changing your work and home environment, exercising, taking proper supplementation, using therapeutic creams and seeing practitioners for complementary wellness visits, you can greatly reduce, and even prevent, the daily throbbing pain of headache and migraine. By following the "Headache Relief Action Plan," inflammation decreases, blood flow increases, muscle loosen, toxins are removed, the mind is relaxed and the body is able to return to its natural state of balance known as homeostasis. While it takes time and effort, and a lifestyle change, you do not have to live your life in debilitating pain just because you have headaches and migraines.

To be honest with you, now at the age of 47, I do find myself with a headache now and again; even bad ones. Why? Because sometimes life gets in the way and outside pressures and triggers turn you around. Because I'm human, I also get complacent and a bit slack in my daily choices. I stay up too late or consume too many food triggers in one day. But the good news is, I know each and every time that I am in control of the headaches and they do not control me. How? Because I can identify in the moment the headache strikes, exactly why it has come, and what type it is. And I know exactly what to do to reduce the pain and symptoms of that specific headache and stop its movement into a bigger, stronger, longer headache. The information in this book, especially the content in the "Headache Relief Action Plan" will show you, too.

The notion that chronic headaches and migraines are a fixture and cannot be cured is one of the biggest myths. If most headaches can be prevented (excluding those that result due to an injury or some other disease), then the cure is found in the methods of prevention. The problem with the Western medical model is that it does not see headaches in a holistic light, and the statistics and data published by the WHO, discussed previously indicate that this approach is not effective. However, traditional and holistic medicines have found natural methods for increasing bone density and regenerating soft tissue. This natural approach to healing and reversing the damage done by headaches and migraines is based on the use of supplements, topical creams and energy medicine. In the chapters that follow, you will learn more about these natural approaches and how they can help you.

MYTH #8
Drugs Are the Only Solution for "Managing" Headaches

This is the biggest myth of all because it is inculcated in the minds of physicians and patients from medical school to prime-time pain-pill product commercials. Over-the-counter and prescription painkillers are effective in providing headache patients with relief, but that doesn't mean they're the only way to treat the pain caused by headaches. Also, these pills treat the pain, the symptom, and do nothing to change the root cause or trigger of the headaches themselves. And so, the headaches return again and again on many other days.

Headache myths are as common as headaches themselves. The only way to debunk these myths is through education and personal experience. If you're not sure if what you believe about headaches is true, consult a headache specialist to confirm. But when you can see the forest for the trees, you will see and feel how changing your lifestyle, environment, choices, actions, thoughts and beliefs can have a tremendous effect on preventing your headaches. This change can also significantly reduce the quantity and severity of your headaches, and restore your quality of life.

Additional Thoughts

It is my sincere wish you do not suffer the many debilitating symptoms of headache and migraine and have your life derailed by them. I hope you brought an open mind to my explanation of why the eight myths do not hold water and you now see why you do not have to remain a prisoner to them. While it may be true that these eight myths are popularly believed, they are not grounded in irrefutable fact. Dismiss these myths and learn the facts so you can change your headache and migraine experience in most cases by preventing the progression of both headaches and migraines. At the same time, you will reduce symptoms and improve your quality of life on a daily basis.

Knowledge is power and understanding fosters wisdom. I recommend the book, *Virus of the Mind* by Richard Brodie. Not only will it help you understand how your beliefs are created but also how to protect yourself from outside forces that can corrupt your mind into believing one thing over another (even when the one thing is not correct or helpful to you).

Chapter 2 will give you a better understanding of where you stand and how to relate to the powerful, potentially life-changing information and action steps provided later in the book.

CHAPTER REVIEW

- Knowledge truly is power; separating truth from myth is essential to begin your journey to a life free from chronic headaches and migraines.
- Many people who suffer from headaches believe headaches are a disease to be managed. They are not. Headaches are symptoms you can manage, reduce and prevent over time.
- You do not have to accept headaches and migraine as a normal part of life.
- You can look healthy, be active, and eat well and still have many triggers for your headaches. You must embrace a holistic lifestyle change.
- You can exercise with headaches and migraines to help reduce the frequency of headache onset.
- You can improve your symptoms through controlling your lifestyle and external environment.
- Your diagnosis does not sentence you to a life devoid of joy and activity.
- You do not have to live in pain; a headache-free life is your birthright. There is hope!
- Your headaches and migraines are symptoms that can be controlled and prevented; I'll show you how.

Cluster
Exertion
Tension
Migraine
Stress
Sleep
Allergy
BioChemicals
Sinus
Oxygen
Diet Rebound
Imbalances
Headache
Exercise

CHAPTER 2

HEADACHE TYPES AND TRIGGERS

Headaches are a complex family of disorders consisting of nearly 30 different classifications. According to the National Headache Foundation's fact sheet:

> "More than 45 million Americans suffer from recurring headaches. That's 32 million more than the number of people who suffer from asthma, diabetes and coronary heart disease combined... Americans spend more than $4 billion each year on over-the-counter pain relief for headaches. Migraine sufferers alone lose more than 157 million workdays to headache and related symptoms each year and other garden-variety headaches are responsible for another 2.8 million lost workdays. Time lost from work and resulting medical expenses due to headaches are estimated to cost American industry $50 billion each year."[1]

These are troubling numbers and the unnecessary suffering from pain and loss in income is staggering. Luckily, the information presented in this book can help people take control of their headaches and drastically reduce those numbers. Could such a movement really take hold? I hope so!

Most medical organizations and headache experts classify headaches into two groups: primary and secondary. As a chronic sufferer and wellness advocate versed in several disciplines, I would disagree with how the medical community views headaches.

According to the accepted medical definition, primary headaches occur without an identifiable cause or underlying condition. They are painful but not serious, and, include such headache types as tension headaches, migraine headaches, cluster headaches, exertion headaches and sex headaches. However, if you understand the full picture of why headaches happen, and acknowledge that lifestyle triggers and external factors contribute to them, and, if you are like me and have suffered chronic mixed headaches for decades and sought advanced education, then you will agree that there is in fact identifiable causes and conditions that trigger headaches.

For example, tension type headaches are caused by stress and tension held in the body, causing restriction of oxygen, blood, and tightness of muscles. Migraine headaches are caused by neurological and blood vessel changes, which themselves have many triggers. Sex headaches are caused by a combination of over exertion, holding of the breath, elevated blood pressure and other things that are known triggers as we will see later in this chapter and in others.

Secondary headaches, by common medical understanding, are potentially life-threatening and do indeed result from specific underlying, biological conditions. Because this classification of headaches is potentially life-taking, and outside the scope of this book, I would like to discuss them briefly before moving on to the more common types of headache that most people experience.

POTENTIALLY LIFE-THREATENING HEADACHES

Headaches that are the result of an underlying biological problem are indeed rare. These are potentially the most lethal, and, must, under all circumstances, be ruled out. Such headaches include those caused by meningitis, encephalitis, brain aneurysm, tumors, diseased blood vessels, concussions, bacterial infections, and other serious disorders.

I would like to share the advice of the National Association of Neurological Disorders and Stroke[2], who warn that if you or a loved one experiences a headache with the following signs, seek immediate medical attention:

- Very sudden, severe headache that may be accompanied by a stiff neck
- Severe headache accompanied by fever, nausea or vomiting that is not related to another illness
- Sudden "worst" headache, often accompanied by confusion, weakness, double vision or loss of consciousness (called a "thunderclap" headache because it occurs suddenly and severely)
- Headache that worsens over days or weeks or has changed in pattern or behavior
- Headache following a head injury
- Headache occurring with a loss of sensation or weakness in any part of the body, which could be a sign of a stroke
- Headache associated with convulsions
- Headache associated with shortness of breath
- New onset of two or more headaches a week

- Persistent headache in someone who has been previously headache-free, particularly someone over age 50
- New headaches in someone with a history of cancer, immune suppression or HIV/AIDS
- Headache that occurs with upright position and goes away when lying flat

Unfortunately, the approach outlined in this book cannot prevent these very serious headaches as their cause is difficult to prevent or account for. These headaches require specialized medical attention.

But, please, don't let this deter you from reading on and implementing the "Headache Relief Action Plan" as part of your new headache-free lifestyle. You see, less than 20% of ALL headaches have a serious, potentially life-threatening component or origin. This means that over 80% of headache and migraine types are preventable.

COMMON HEADACHE TYPES

If you suffer chronic headaches or even acute headaches or migraines several times per year, then the chances are that your headaches are not of the above described life-threatening nature. So, read on and get to know more about some of the different types of headaches, risk factors, and triggers. This knowledge will help you along your headache-free path and help you make more sense out of the plans of action outlined here. Let's now look at the most common headache types.

Tension Type Headaches (TTH)

Tension Type Headaches (TTH) are the most common types of headache, accounting for approximately 90% of all headaches. They are usually episodic and their root cause is easily identifiable.

I prefer to refer to them as "muscle contraction headaches," as they are caused by excessive muscle tension in the head, neck and shoulders that irritate the trigeminal nerve, causing pain.

Muscle contraction headaches are classified as either chronic (repeated) or episodic (sporadic), and generally last anywhere from a few minutes to a few hours or even several days. They are symptomatically characterized by a stiff neck and shoulders and a dull, achy pain in the head, temples and forehead that feels as if a band were being tightened around the head.

While annoying, these headaches do not necessarily hamper daily life functions, and, for those who are prone to them, can be triggered by a great many things, including stress and anxiety, eye strain, poor posture, forward head posture, structural misalignment (including TMJ), and sleep deprivation. Tension headaches tend to quickly subside after the trigger is resolved.

Exertion Headaches

Exertion headaches are also quite common among those who are susceptible to getting headaches. These can either be triggered by sudden spurts of energy or prolonged use of muscles. Exertion headaches bring throbbing or pounding pain but are often short in duration. They generally occur when one sits up too quickly after lying prone for some time, or after a strenuous exertion when lifting or pushing a heavy object, straining while going to the bathroom or during sexual intercourse. In other words, abdominal contraction combined with the holding of the breath and physical exertion can cause exertion headaches.

Strenuous activity like heavy lifting or moving without properly warming up also stresses the muscles and oxygen circulation because of restricted breathing and tightening of the muscles. Exertion headache pain is a result of blood vessels in the head and scalp expanding due to of swelling in the arteries and veins.

Stress Headaches

Mental and emotional stress causes negative effects on the liver, digestion, and respiration. Such psychological distress, even for a short period of time, includes a racing mind, obsessive thoughts, unending worry, muscle tension and spasm, poor appetite or too great an appetite, digestive disorders, constipation, insomnia, poor blood flow, belabored breathing, neck and shoulder tension, and the possible onset or continuation of bad habits such as dependence on alcohol, drugs, pain killers, food and caffeine. Any one of these things by itself can trigger any number of different types of headaches. But when these forces of antagonism are combined (as they generally are when triggered by stress), the headache problem can become chronic and insufferable.

Migraine Headaches

Migraine headaches are the bane of existence of those who suffer these debilitating and life-wrecking events. One in 10 Americans suffer from them. Migraines are no ordinary headaches and are not caused by tension, stress or allergies, like many other types of headaches, but are actually related to neurological (nerve) and vascular (blood vessel) changes.

Vasoconstriction and vasodilation cause extreme pain – and, often, an aura before migraine onset — along with sensitivity to light, smell and sound. Luckily, true migraines affect only one in 10 Americans (10% of people worldwide, but three times as many women as men).

Chronic migraine headaches are not only incapacitating, they are traumatic events in the lives of headache sufferers.

Migraine headaches are of the vascular type, as they are believed to be associated with the constriction and expansion of blood vessels in the head and are categorized as either *classic* or *common*. Classic migraines are usually associated with the presence of a view-obstructing aura some 30 minutes or so prior to an attack. Common migraines are not accompanied or preceded by an aura, but are no less painful.

Migraine sufferers usually describe their pain as throbbing or pounding on one side of the head in tandem with their pulse, which changes to a steady sharp or blinding pain with numbness in the affected area and featuring general somatic weakness. Attacks usually last for as short as several hours or as long as three or more days, and are generally accompanied by trembling, sweating and vomiting. During attacks, sufferers tend to be hypersensitive to light, sounds and smells and often desire to be left alone in a quiet room with the blankets pulled over their head, and ice packs on their temples.

Migraines are now recognized as a neurological disorder. Attacks begin when the central nervous system is exposed to an environment which provokes, or "triggers" a migraine, causing neurochemical changes. External factors can include chemical smells, flickering lights, and atmospheric conditions, among others.

Studies show that those who experience the so-called "classic migraine" (that is, the migraine that follows a visual aura) have elevated levels of homocysteine. Homocysteine is an amino acid in the blood that, when it rises too high, can lead to a host of health issues, including blood vessel blockages and migraine headaches.

Levels of homocysteine rise when it is not metabolized properly; this can be caused by low levels of certain B vitamins and folic acid. Studies have shown that in addition to diets high in these vitamins, or merely supplementing with B12, B6 and folate, you can help the body process and metabolize homocysteine and bring it down to a normal level, thus helping prevent classic migraines. A blood test can determine if high levels of homocysteine is causing your migraines.

Cluster Headaches

While they are less common than migraines, cluster headaches are without doubt the most painful and difficult to deal with, affecting roughly one million Americans, 90% of them male.

Cluster headaches have vascular origins. Changes in blood vessel size and pressure (known as vasoconstriction and vasodilation) is the cause of the pain, which tends to occur in a "cluster" of time and linger over the course of days or even months. The pain associated with this headache is generally "clustered" around the temple or behind one eye or temple area and is often described as sharp and piercing and also includes symptoms like tearing and nasal congestion, reddening of the affected eye, and sweating. Unlike migraines, cluster headaches do not occur with nausea, vomiting or sensitivity to light; although, in my experience, when accompanied with a migraine, death feels like the only option.

While the direct cause of cluster headaches is not certain, research supports the theory that they may originate in the hypothalamus. It is in this part of the brain that levels of neurotransmitter production are affected. Inadequate levels of the feel-good neurotransmitter serotonin are a known headache trigger as are changes of season and temperature, certain foods, caffeine, alcohol, too little or too much sleep, hunger or overeating, changes in blood sugar and blood fat levels, food or chemical allergies, seasonal allergies and constipation. All of these are related to lifestyle and fully "fixable" by implementing the "Headache Relief Action Plan!"

Sinus/Allergy/Sensitivity Headaches

Once upon a time, doctors associated migraines with allergies and also misdiagnosed them as sinus headaches, since they share common symptoms. While both suppositions have since been disproved, many secondary headaches have an underlying food, chemical or environmental allergy or sensitivity at their root.

For those prone to getting them, triggers for allergy/sensitivity headaches can include stress, food, light, cigarette smoke, fabric softener, alcohol, pesticides, pollen—almost anything. Pain associated with allergy headaches is generally dull and diffused over the entire head, with no easily identifiable location. Such headaches are known to come on several hours after contact with the problematic substance, and are easy to offset by simply removing the thing to which the allergic reaction was caused.

When the sinuses are inflamed, nasal passages narrow. This leads to pressure in the sinus cavities and provides a place for viral and bacterial infections to grow. This can lead to sensitivity and throbbing pain around the cheeks, nose and eye areas. This is where the link to sinus derives and why most over-the-counter medication for this type of headache falls under the name "sinus/allergy relief." The prevention program outlined in this book can prevent these sinus/allergy/sensitivity headaches from ruining your life again.

Rebound/Recuperative Headaches

Rebound or recuperative headaches occur as the body "rebounds" from over-consumption or withdrawal from too many analgesics or prescription medications, too much coffee or caffeine beverages, elevated adrenaline levels, sleep disorders, and the like.

Like cluster headaches, rebound headaches are vascular in nature and are thus characterized by steady pounding or throbbing on one or both sides of the head caused by constricting and dilating blood vessels. This type of vascular headache is in theory the easiest to prevent, but since it is directly triggered by poor lifestyle choices, it may be the most difficult to eliminate.

In essence, rebound headaches are a recuperative measure carried out by the body, telling you something is wrong and forcing rest and change in behavior by bringing on severe head pain. See the following chapter on how prescription pain medication actually causes headaches!

COMMON HEADACHE TRIGGERS

You now have basic knowledge that there are many different types and categories of headaches. You also know that you don't necessarily get the same type of headache every time, and, oftentimes, they attack in combination, which is why Advil diminishes the pain sometimes and not at other times. It also explains why a chiropractic adjustment alleviates your headache today but not tomorrow.

An in-depth look at the most infamous headache triggers and how they can be removed or prevented is presented in the following chapters. Let's take a quick look at an overview of the headache spectrum.

Mild Oxygen Deprivation

Oxygen is the most vital element you need to live. Yet, while the atmosphere offers us an ample oxygen supply, we neglect to put it to best use, rarely filling our lungs. We take quick short breaths and compromise our health. Mild oxygen deprivation causes headaches, and also generalized chronic pain syndromes. Caused by poor breathing or breath obstruction, this is one of the hidden, yet most direct, preventable causes of headaches.

Mild Dehydration

With the abundance of water available and the sheer necessity of it for the betterment of our health and well-being, it is a wonder that the many illnesses and ailments—including chronic headaches—are actually triggered by people being in a chronic state of mild dehydration. As the water content of tissues falls to a certain point due to dehydration, the bi-layer membranes that surround cells contract, forming a barrier that prevents further water loss. This occurrence obstructs the free movement of molecules, so that metabolism and elimination are limited. Slow metabolism and elimination leads to build-up of toxins in the blood, which can manifest as headaches and migraines.

Improper Biochemical Levels

For the body to function at homeostasis, all its chemicals and hormones must be at proper levels. However, when levels of certain chemicals drop or rise, they can trigger various types of headaches. Low levels of the neurotransmitter serotonin, high levels of fats in the blood, low blood sugar, high levels of histamine, low levels of magnesium and vitamins A, B and C are all known headache triggers. Regulating these chemicals in the body and maintaining those levels is a key factor to preventing certain types of headaches.

Food and Chemical Sensitivities

For people who are prone to them, headaches resulting from food, chemical and environmental sensitivities or allergies can become a chronic problem. The chemicals found in the tap water we drink and the pesticide residues and hormones in the foods we eat can trigger headaches. Specific types of foods, such as aged cheese, red wine, tomato sauce, pickled foods, dairy products, cocoa, alcohol and caffeine are known culprits. Learning how to avoid the sensitivities and changing eating habits will do much to eliminating those triggers.

Sleep Deprivation

Sleep deprivation is a sure trigger of headaches. Anxiety, stress, digestive issues, consuming alcohol at night, and low levels of serotonin can lead to poor sleeping patterns. Proper, sound sleep happens in distinct stages, and these stages regulate the deep tissue healing of our muscles, relax the nervous systems, and regulate hormones and help reestablish homeostasis. Improper restorative rest after exercise or long weeks of stress-laden work, general insomnia or the inability to sleep straight through the night do much to trigger both migraine headaches and muscle-contraction (tension-type) headaches.

Inadequate Exercise

Endorphins are the body's natural pain killers and they are released during prolonged physical activity. One of the major causes of headaches is inactivity. Aside from lowering oxygen intake and endorphin levels in the body, a host of other diseases result from lack of exercise. A sedentary lifestyle also assists in the creation of imbalances in the musculoskeletal system, which can also trigger certain types of headaches. And for those who do exercise, or don't but who are workaholics, inadequate rest and sleep can also cause headaches through not allowing the body to rejuvenate itself.

Musculoskeletal Imbalances

Imbalances in both the muscular and skeletal systems can lead to headaches in a number of ways. Misaligned vertebrae can pinch nerves, sending pain signals to the head. Nerve sensitivity and muscle spasms in the back, shoulders and neck can cause muscle-contraction or tension-type headaches. Improper posture while seated or standing, ergonomically incorrect positions when typing or playing the piano, for example, also lead to musculoskeletal imbalances that can trigger headaches. When combined with even moderate exercise and postural correction, proper stretching and progressive antagonistic exercises can correct such imbalances to the musculoskeletal system and prevent such triggers from causing headaches.

Chronic Stress and Psychosomatic Triggers

The effects of stress include nail biting, anxiety, a racing mind, obsessive thoughts, compulsive behavior, unending worry, muscle tension and spasm, poor appetite or too great an appetite, digestive disorders, constipation, insomnia, poor blood flow, belabored breathing, neck pain, shoulder tension and the possible onset or continuation of bad habits such as dependence on alcohol, drugs, painkillers, food and caffeine. Any one of these things by itself can trigger any number of different headache types.

PLEASE KNOW THERE IS HOPE!

For me, the worst part about headache and migraine is that many who have it believe there is no hope for them. They think that because they have headaches and migraines today, they will have it tomorrow. They think that because they experience excruciating pain today, they will experience it tomorrow and keep experiencing it for the rest of their life. It is as if the trajectory of headaches and migraines to them is inevitable; and, therefore, there is no hope. This does not have to be the case. Nothing about headaches and migraines is "inevitable" if you understand the condition and take steps to control it.

Even though this is the case, many don't know or believe it because of what they have been told. As a result, many headache and migraine centers report that a full one-half (50 percent) of Americans suffering with headaches and migraines do not believe anything can be done to help ease their pain. Why? Because the drug-based therapies they have been following are not useful in providing a change to the condition – only symptomatic relief. Yes, immediate relief of pain is a good thing, and, certainly, drugs are the fastest means for that relief. However, there are two problems with relying on synthetic drug therapies over the long term:

Problem 1: The drugs and cortisone injections are toxic to the system, causing in some cases damage to the liver and stomach lining, weakening of the joint cartilage and the immune system, and GI tract issues.

Problem 2: Drugs do not change the course of the condition, and, thus, as the headache and migraine worsens over time, drugs that are more potent are needed, causing more toxicity and potentially damaging side effects.

As such, the reliance on drug therapies cause damage to other parts of the body, and require constant increases in dose, further tearing apart your system (see Chapter 3). The end result is little, lasting relief with greater health consequences.

The good news is that a multi-pronged approach to headache and migraine prevention, like the "Headache Relief Action Plan," can do wonders and even feel like a miracle to those suffering its nasty symptoms. Because there is no cure, it is extremely important to become proactive in managing, treating and slowing down the condition. I will say again that by reading this book in the order it is presented, you will gain knowledge and insight into headaches and migraines. This will provide you with understanding and hope. From this, you will be more motivated to approach the various natural solutions and make the necessary lifestyle changes in your life to improve the quality of your life. *There is hope, and hope is where change begins.*

CHAPTER REVIEW

- More than 45 million Americans suffer headaches, but you don't "have to."

- Less than 20% of all headaches are potentially dangerous with serious side effects. These types are generally acute and sudden and not of the chronic type that this program addresses.

- You can prevent chronic headaches, regardless of their label or type.

- You can take steps to reduce the onset, duration, frequency and pain level of headaches now. It is within your grasp to do so.

- Drug-based therapies set you on a path to worsening health without addressing the real cause of your headaches and migraines.

- You can reduce and then prevent your headaches and migraines with the "Headache Action Plan" – starting now.

CHAPTER 3

HOW MAINSTREAM MEDICINE CAN MAKE HEADACHES WORSE

The future of prescription headache medication is said to hold the promise of mind-boggling progress. The amount of research and development being done today by pharmaceutical, med-tech and bio-tech companies is staggering.

There's just one problem: Medical progress comes at too high a price. It will never be cheap to treat chronic illnesses the high-tech way. In fact, medication for certain disorders can be so expensive that even the most generous HMO or health insurer will cut off sufferers after a year or two.

The American health care system will always be stressed by the high costs of pharmaceuticals, extended hospital stays, and sky-high insurance costs. It's the chronically ill who incur the lion's share of these costs over a long period of time. In many cases, that care can relieve and treat symptoms, but it often cannot provide a cure or prevent the pain and suffering.

It's truly amazing that despite the advances in medical science, an astonishing 25 million Americans suffer migraines and a whopping 9 out of 10 suffer other headaches as part of their daily lives!

These headaches are accepted as inevitable parts of life, and sufferers swallow prescription drugs as a matter of habit, just as they brush their teeth without giving the action a second thought. The problem is chronic headaches and migraines take their toll, not only on the body's ability to maintain a state of homeostasis or wellness, but on the ability to think logically, see clearly, and to feel and act appropriately. The impact all this has on one's quality of life is shattering: jobs lost, relationships ruined, motivation diminished, and happiness disintegrated.

Our habitual response on getting headaches is to swallow over-the-counter (OTC) analgesics and anti-inflammatory drugs or prescription medications. Time has undeniably shown that these do not provide long-term headache relief. In fact, while pain-relieving drugs are mainstays of many chronic headache management programs, their long-term use adversely affects the digestive tract, liver and kidneys through toxic build-up. This, of course, leads to taking more and more OTC analgesics, which lead to rebound headaches, which in turn lead to taking stronger prescriptions medications. This vicious circle continues until the pain goes from once in a while to becoming a chronic problem. This makes the headache problem not only worse, but far more difficult to treat and eliminate.

Despite their popularity and first-line use due to their fast-acting analgesic properties, nonsteroidal anti-inflammatory drugs (NSAIDs) are a mainstay of chronic-pain management. The *New England Journal of Medicine* cautions against their side effects:

"Long-term use of prescription and over-the-counter nonsteroidal anti-inflammatory drugs (NSAIDs), such as Ibuprofen, can adversely affect a person's digestive tract, liver and kidneys."[1]

A study from the University of Pennsylvania Medical Center found that some of the new NSAIDs approved by the FDA might increase the risk of heart attacks, strokes and other harmful cardiovascular problems. Additionally, almost all NSAIDs can cause serious gastrointestinal side effects – including ulceration, bleeding and perforation – at any time and without warning. Not to mention, their link to a greater risk of cardiovascular (heart) problems and possible gastrointestinal (stomach and intestine) issues. When it comes to drugs, there are just so many options… and none of them healthy. Let's look at why this is.

Acetaminophen

While acetaminophen (Tylenol) offers temporary pain relief and fever reduction, it does not reduce swelling (inflammation). It can be harmful to the liver and kidney if you take more than the recommended dose.

Non-Steroidal Anti-inflammatory Drugs (NSAIDs)

NSAIDs work fast to relieve acute pain, but they may also cause gastrointestinal bleeding. They can also be harmful if you have high blood pressure or kidney disease. And they should NEVER be given to children. Aspirin has been associated with the onset of a children's disease called Reye's syndrome.

COX-2 Inhibitors

Yes, these work as well as NSAIDs and are less harsh on the stomach, but numerous reports of heart attacks and stroke have prompted the FDA to re-evaluate the risks and benefits of the

COX-2s. COX-2 drugs such as Vioxx and Celebrex were actually taken off the market because of these risks.

Opioid Narcotics

Opioid (narcotic) analgesics are derived from or related to opium. They bind to opioid receptors, which present in many regions of the nervous system and are involved in pain signaling and control. This class of drug includes fentanyl (Actiq, Duragesic, Fentora), hydrocodone (Hysingla ER, Zohydro ER), hydrocodone/acetaminophen (Lorcet, Lortab, Norco, Vicodin), hydromorphone (Dilaudid, Exalgo), meperidine (Demerol), methadone (Dolophine, Methadose), morphine (Astramorph, Avinza, Kadian, MS Contin, Ora-Morph SR), oxycodone (OxyContin, Oxecta, Roxicodone), oxycodone and acetaminophen (Percocet, Endocet, Roxicet), and oxycodone and naloxone (Targiniq ER). I am sure as a chronic migraine or headache sufferer, you have been prescribed one or more of these drugs over time.

These narcotic drugs are very powerful and do cover the pain, temporarily. Yet, they are highly addictive and have serious side effects. In fact, according to the Centers for Disease Control and Prevention (CDCP), between 2014 and 2015, deaths from synthetic opioids, including fentanyl, increased a by a shocking 72.2%. According to the CDCP report, synthetic opioid use resulted in the following:

> *"Synthetic opioid deaths increased in 16 states... Deaths from so-called natural opioids, which include the prescription medications morphine and codeine, and semi-synthetic opioids, which include the prescription drugs oxycodone and hydrocodone, decreased 2.6% from 2014 to 2015. However, they are still responsible for more than 12,700 deaths."*[2]

REBOUND HEADACHES LINKED TO ANALGESICS & OPIOIDS

If death and addiction were not bad enough, analgesics and opioids are linked to a higher risk rebound headache when compared with other treatments. Kristian Thorlund, PhD and colleagues of McMaster University in Ontario, Canada, studied the effects of rebound headaches tied to drugs, also known as medication-overuse headaches (MOH). Their study was published in the *Journal of Headache and Pain*, and found several alarming conclusions:

> *"Our study suggests that in patients with acute episodic migraine, the rate of MOH associated with analgesics and opioids is considerably higher than the rate of MOH associated with triptans and ergots...These findings provide incentives for better monitoring of use of analgesics and opioids for treating acute migraine, and suggest possible clinical preference for use of so-called 'migraine-specific' treatments, that is, triptans and ergots."*[3]

THE GOLDEN RULE OF PAIN

When experiencing pain, and deciding whether or not to reach for OTC or Rx drugs, please keep in mind that pain and inflammation are not the biggest problem. The biggest problem is simply that **Drugs Don't Heal.** Why? Because headaches and migraines are not caused by a deficiency of drugs. If you are suffering chronic headaches and migraines, please repeat this mantra:

Drugs don't fix the problem.
Drugs only mask the symptoms.
Pain and inflammation are symptoms, not diseases.

Many who follow only the mainstream medical approach to headache and migraine end up with rebound headaches, addictions, organ damage, and even death—and the headaches remain ever present. I didn't want this for myself and I don't want this for you. And you don't want this either. Again, let me say that the medications may help in the short run, and may be necessary to get through your days, but they fall short over time and have serious side effects. Please keep an open mind.

When it comes to embracing a natural and all-encompassing headache and migraine solution, chemical pain relief medications should only be used temporarily, and as needed for breakthrough symptoms while ramping up the natural approach presented in this book. The more natural and preventive approach is to understand the pain problem, and take proactive approaches to relieving pain and preventing new pain.

And there are so many options to choose for headache and migraine relief.

I know I mentioned this in the previous chapter. However, I did so to reinforce how something as simple and natural as a particular supplement or meditative exercise has been proven – in a clinical setting – to be a powerful solution in overcoming chronic headache conditions that mainstream medicine has given up on trying to cure. This natural treatment approach, along with the realization of the dangers of continuous prescription drug use, should give you hope and motivation to commit to the "Headache Relief Action Plan." The plan is worth the lifestyle changes required to improve your condition and your quality of life.

CHOOSE LIFESTYLE CHANGES OVER DRUGS!

Natural, lasting drug-free pain relief is based on wide reaching lifestyle changes. Simple changes can go a long way to reduce and prevent pain in your life.

It is important to know that a headache is not a disease; it is a symptom. I know I keep repeating myself, but I want you to understand this important point fully. Make it your mantra so you can proceed in the full belief that prevention of headaches is, without a doubt, within your personal grasp. Something or several things are needed to trigger a headache. Thus, while taking pain medication can certainly decrease the pain or other symptoms, they will not prevent the triggers from causing the headache. Controlling for triggers leads to prevention of headaches.

Again, the majority of things that cause or trigger headaches are the result of our lifestyles. When we choose to indulge in the foods, beverages and activities that are known triggers of headaches, we choose to give ourselves a headache.

We then choose to take a pain-relieving medication to stop the headache instead of changing our behaviors that maintain our unhealthy lifestyle. That may sound harsh, but it is true. And believe me, having suffered excruciating headaches for decades, I know that we don't feel like headaches are a choice. And sometime they are not. But for the common headaches not related to diseases or tumors or traumatic injury, the prevention of them is a choice worth choosing.

So how does lifestyle trigger headaches? In many ways, all of them are related to our daily choices and behaviors.

Most headaches can be controlled as long as we choose a proactive approach rather than a reactive one. Lifestyle triggers include the duration and quality of our sleep, our work methods, exercise habits, emotional states, and stress-relieving abilities. Other triggers include our diet and the environment in the home and workplace.

We will look at how to work around all of these triggers, and, if it seems confusing or daunting, don't worry a bit. If you follow the "Headache Relief Action Plan" provided in Part Three of this book, it will all be taken care of for you!

CHAPTER REVIEW

- Mainstream medicine offers short-term relief, and can actually make your headache and migraine worse… it creates a new, additional, "rebound headache" for you.
- Many medical doctors throw elaborate and costly procedures at this growing national health emergency – all with little to show for it.
- Don't fall victim to the medical myth that you must depend on others for your care.
- Golden Rule of Pain: Drugs don't heal; they mask symptoms. You deserve better.
- Prescription and over-the-counter drugs are far from safe; they wreak havoc on vital organs without addressing the cause of your pain.
- Pain medications can help temporarily as you step on the road to natural relief from chronic headaches and migraines with the "Headache Relief Action Plan." But, you will need to use them less and less as you progress with the program each week.

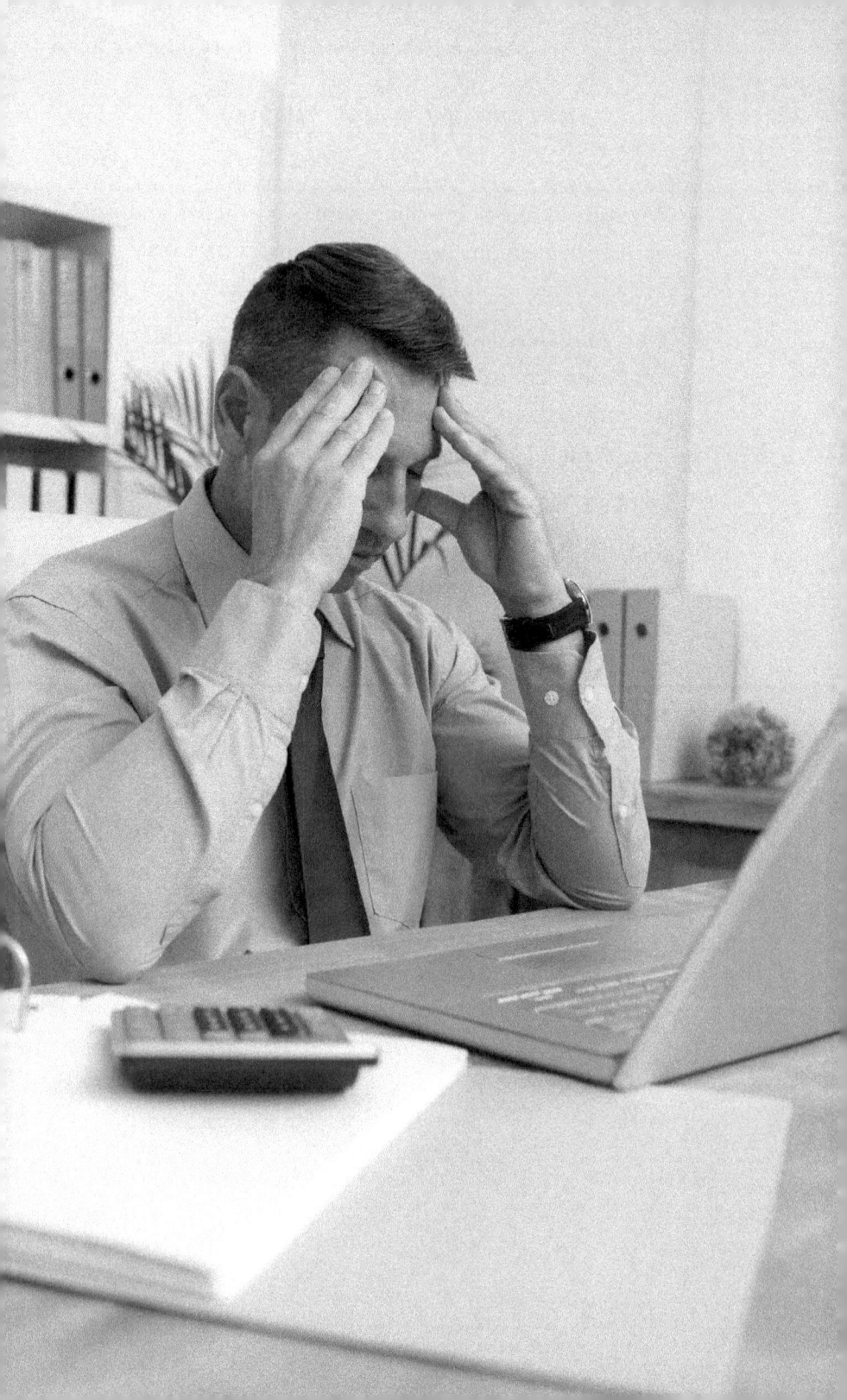

CHAPTER 4

THE 15 BIGGEST HEADACHE MISTAKES PEOPLE MAKE

We all make mistakes; it's part of the human condition. We all also have bad habits in our lives that seem to be things we do on auto-pilot without much thought. When it comes to stopping headaches and migraines — especially chronic ones — you need to correct the mistakes that trigger them and live each day by making decisions *on purpose*, instead of letting habit direct you. It is important to be *in charge* of your choices, actions and behaviors if you really want to put an end to your headaches.

It is to be expected you will make mistakes when it comes to identifying and dealing with your headaches and migraines or in helping a loved one manage his or her headaches. This chapter will help you identify the most commonly made mistakes. However, many people don't realize they are making mistakes, and this can lead to real problems for headache sufferers: the condition changes from acute to chronic, and the daily choices on what to do about it only make the problem worse. Any little success is derailed.

If the definition of insanity is doing the same things over and over again while expecting different results, why do we continue to look at and treat headaches in the same way? When it comes to headaches and migraines, some things work well, others fall short, and others make the situation worse. Doing the same things, and making the same mistakes repeatedly will definitely not get you to the place you need to be.

Now we are going to go over what I see to be the 15 most common mistakes people make when dealing with headaches and migraines. Please read them over and see what resonates with you. Then, let them go and move on and start looking toward positive change by embracing a new way of doing things and implementing the "Headache Relief Action Plan," explained in detail later in this book.

The mistakes people often make in relation to headaches and migraines are rooted in three common areas: 1) inaction, 2) misinformation, and 3) giving up. Let's take a look at these now.

⊕ MISTAKES OF INACTION ⊕

MISTAKE #1
Thinking You Don't Need to See a Doctor About Headaches

While it is true that a very small percentage of headaches require medical attention, it's a mistake to think you don't need to seek medical attention at certain times. These exceptions include cases where a headache comes on following a fall or blow to the head; having a "sudden onset" headache seemingly out of nowhere; and, experiencing "the worst headache in your life" when you don't usually get them.

I'd like to repeat the warning that appears in the front of this book to alert and remind you when it may be necessary to seek medical attention for your headaches. The National Institute of Neurological Disorders and Stroke (NINDS) suggest you should seek prompt medical care if you experience any of the following symptoms:

- An abrupt, severe headache or a sudden headache associated with a stiff neck
- A headache associated with fever or convulsions or accompanied by confusion or loss of consciousness
- A headache following a blow to the head or associated with pain in the eye or ear
- Persistent headache in a person who was previously headache-free
- Recurring headaches in children

The good news is that most, nearly 90%, of headaches are benign; painful and debilitating, but not potentially life-threatening

MISTAKE #2
Waiting Too Long to Address Your Headaches

Because many believe headaches are harmless or there is nothing that can be done about them, it is not uncommon for people to ignore them. I am here to tell you that waiting too long to take charge of your headaches is a huge mistake. People wait too long to address their headaches both at the onset of a single headache episode or in response to getting headaches frequently. Here's why this is a mistake.

For any treatment to work at its strongest, it must be applied at first sign of a headache. That means the moment you see an aura, feel a tinge of pain in your head, or experience any other warning sign that usually precedes your headaches, you must take action. Even strong prescription medication, like triptans, are much less effective and often do not work once the headache has "taken hold." And the gentler, natural remedies and procedures shared in this book must be employed as close as possible to the "first signs" of an oncoming headache. When you wait to employ the emergency pain-relief techniques taught in this book or wait to take pain medications like Excedrin, they are less effective and result in greater consumption and reliance on them.

Another mistake of waiting too long is to acknowledge when headaches change from being "now and then" to becoming a chronic fixture in your life. The thing is people don't realize they are having frequent headaches because they kind of sneak up on you. Everybody is popping pills for pain and allergies and diseases so frequently that even the repeated taking of Aspirin, Excedrin, Ibuprofen and other over the counter (OTC) medications seems normal. It is not normal or safe to take pain-relieving drugs on a daily, weekly or regular basis. The sooner you notice your headaches have increased in frequency or duration… the better your chances of identifying their underlying causes or triggers.

In both cases mentioned here, once you experience the first sign of headache begin, and, once you realize or have been diagnosed with chronic headaches or migraines, you must become highly proactive in managing, treating, and preventing them. Reduction of symptoms and changes in lifestyle are essential from the start. It often takes quite a bit of discipline to realize that changing your life (how you work, exercise, eat, etc.) is needed when it comes to overcoming the debilitating nature of this condition. Waiting too long to do something about headaches and migraines is a mistake.

Waiting too long or ignoring your headaches is the biggest mistakes you can make because it allows the condition to take hold and entrench itself in the body, progress and wreak havoc. Waiting allows headaches and migraines to steal days and joy from your life. There is no time like the present. Make the decision to begin the rest of your life today by taking control of your headache and migraine condition.

MISTAKE #3
Not Doing Anything Because You Think Migraines Don't Last Long

This mistake is an extension of the above mistake of waiting too long to address your headaches and taking back control of your life. Many who experience headaches don't want to take medicine and don't think they need to do something else to stop the pain because they believe it will only last an hour or two.

The truth is that migraines generally last from between 72 hours (3 days) to a week or longer. Mine used to be up to 8 days in a row at times. And, depending on the external environment and your internal state (stress, sleep, water, food, etc.), other types of headaches can last for days. What's worse, one type of headache can trigger another type. For example, a sinus headache can trigger a tension headaches which can then trigger a migraine.

It is a mistake to think you don't have to respond to a headache at first sign because you think it won't last long and nothing needs to be done. If you get headaches semi-frequently or have them chronically, you especially need to correct this mistake and avoid waiting. The faster you respond, the less needs to be done to stop the headache before it has had a chance to "set in." Conversely, the longer you wait, the stronger the approach and the less effective any approach to the pain relief will be. This is especially true of pain-relieving medication, and is why you need to take more and more, and end up jumping from OTC to prescription meds over time. And this can lead to rebound headaches as well as liver and kidney damage.

Do not let the waiting mistake make your headaches worse, increase their frequency and duration, or allow them to ruin your body. Once you feel a headache begin or sense a headache coming on, do something about it right away. Do not delay!

MISTAKE #4
Not Taking Action Because Headaches Don't Affect Your Quality of Life

It is so easy to ignore problems in life, especially those around our health and wellness. After all, we have so much on our plates with work, school, the kids, familial obligations; who has time for self-care? Also, we have many health issues and headaches are just one of the many, so what's the big deal? Life goes on.

Yes, it is true that life goes on for those with pain, illness and disease, but at what quality? Headaches and migraines take their toll and ruin lives. They rob you of your spirit, take the joy out of life, prevent certain activities from being done or enjoyed, and they take time from work and reduce productivity. In short, headaches reduce quality of life little by little and then suddenly as if all at once, your life is a shadow of what it once was. You no longer exercise. You are on a handful of medication for chronic pain. You can't go out socially or must return early from a night out because the pain becomes so severe.

It is a mistake to think that headaches are a normal part of life and do not affect your quality of life. Quality of life and a pain-free life is your birthright, and it is a mistake to think otherwise or accept something different. I urge you to take headaches and migraines seriously as enemies that will alter your life for the worse if you don't take control of them now and prevent their future return. Please follow the guidelines in this book.

MISTAKE #5
Not Taking Personal Control of Your Headaches

The most powerful thing you can ever come to know is the fact that no one cares about your headache and migraine conditions as much as you do. Others simply do not have as big a stake in it. You are the one suffering, not them. Relying on healthcare providers to take care of your condition is a big mistake.

You must take personal control of your headaches and migraines. It is only you who can change your lifestyle, and remove the things that negatively affect your health and wellness. It is only you who can eat right, take supplements, and administer pain relieving creams and gels. It is only you who can stretch, walk, exercise, and meditate. So please find a way to become self-empowered and take control. I know it is hard. I struggle with it, too. But if you don't do it, who will? And to help you find that passion for change and develop a self-empowered spirit, I have included material on motivation toward the end of the book. You can do it. I know you can!

✠ MISTAKES OF MISINFORMATION ✠

MISTAKE #6
Only Certain Types of People Get Migraines

When I was growing up with severe headaches, I was led to believe a lot of things that were not true. One of them was that only certain types of people of a specific gender, age, and personality got migraines. And so, my bad headaches were related to allergies or sinus issues and were treated as such with injections and medication. What a mistake it was to believe such nonsense!

The fact is that anyone can experience a migraine and it's a big mistake to believe otherwise. You should not dismiss the idea that you or your child may be having a migraine just because they are more common in women (18%) than men (6%), and more diagnosed in adults than in children (a reflection of the mistake that only adults get migraines). In fact, according to the Migraine Research Foundation, 10% of children experience migraines. What's more, they report that "12% of the population suffers from migraine" and that "migraine is the third most prevalent illness in the world."[1]

Moreover, it is true there is a "headache personality" in people who have a "Type-A" personality. These people are more prone to certain types of headaches. Yet, these are specific headache types triggered by lifestyle choices and behaviors closely associated with that personality (as we'll learn later in the book). But, this slice of the headache pie does not exclude other adults or children from having migraines.

Research indicates that migraines in particular are triggered by neurological changes, which can occur to anyone at any age. It is a mistake to think you are not the right gender, age or personality type to get migraines, and thus avoid having them diagnosed or take action steps, like those outlined in this book, to reduce your pain and eventually prevent them.

MISTAKE #7
Thinking People Outgrow Their Headaches

This is another one of those big misinformation mistakes that are perpetuated by healthcare providers who don't understand headaches and migraines and are at a loss to effectively treat them. It is not uncommon for physicians who are presented with children or teenagers with chronic headaches to say "take these meds as needed and don't worry, they will grow out of them." It seems odd that rather than look for a root cause of the headaches in children and teens, people are led to mistakenly believe that "only adults get headaches" and be told by physicians that their child will "outgrow" them.

This mistake is widespread and a simple "get out of jail free" card for practitioners who are unsuccessful in helping younger people overcome their headaches with medication. Please stop believing this. But know that it is true that many youngsters do stop having headaches as they get older, but not because they "grew out of them." The real reason they stop is because the youngster started making different lifestyle choices. Often this is unconscious and so the mistaken belief is perpetuated.

You see, lifestyle choices both trigger and prevent headaches depending on what you choose. As a child or teen, you have less control over your personal choices because many are made by your parents, such as bed time, what is eaten at meals, what laundry detergent is used, if there is a smoker in the home or chemical rug cleaners applied, and so on. Here's a fun personal example from my own childhood. My mom was not a good cook but she loved us and wanted our food to taste good so she covered our chicken, salads, and veggies with a popular seasoning mix. Of course, that brand, like many on the market back then and today, contained MSG (monosodium glutamate), which is a nasty migraine trigger. She also liked to feed us hot dogs and send us to school with bologna sandwiches, both of which contain migraine triggering nitrates. To make things worse, she was a smoker and second-hand smoke causes headaches along with the strong chemicals she used to mop the kitchen floor. And so, for no fault of my own as a youngster, decisions were being made about my food (MSG and nitrates) and air (smoke and chemicals) that were among the root causes (or triggers) of my migraines. When I became a teenager, and spent more time outside the home, the frequency and duration of my migraines receded. Not because I "grew out of them," but because my environment (smoke, chemicals) changed and my diet (less MSG and nitrates) changed due to doing different things.

It is a mistake to think you or anyone else will simply grow out of their headaches. Choose to educate yourself about the many causes and triggers of headaches and migraines in order to make informed changes to prevent them from recurring now.

MISTAKE #8
Not Acknowledging the Big Role Diet Plays in Headaches

It took a long time for naturalists to gain some respect in America. We've been saying for decades, especially since the 1960s, that diet is essential to health and well-being. Yet, the medical profession wanted nothing to do with this idea, and wrongly asserted that it did not matter what you put in your mouth. Now after decades of tests and discovering that cholesterol, and the fat stored in your body is the home of toxins, and that certain foods change the quality of blood vessels and hormones, the medical experts are changing their stance. You should too, because it is a mistake to believe that diet and nutrition do not play a role in headaches and migraines.

One of the key components of headache and migraine prevention is embracing an organic, nutrient-dense diet and taking nutritional supplements to reduce symptoms and shore up wellness. Since our bodies are created from the stuff we eat, our cells, blood, tissues, nerves, and muscles are formed and reformed every seven years based on the quality of our nutritional intake. And when it comes to reducing symptoms, taking natural supplements to reduce inflammation and ease pain and improve nerve impulse and blood quality is gentler on the body than taking chemicals and artificial drugs.

Diet is among the most common triggers for chronic headaches and migraines. It is also among the most easily addressed. So please, don't fall victim to the diet and nutrition mistake. Instead, embrace the advice given in this book, and be proactive about putting good things into your body.

MISTAKE #9
Thinking Doctors and Medical Specialists Have All the Answers

Americans are taught to believe in a healthcare system based on two categories: generalists and specialists. They are taught to see their primary care physician (i.e., "family doctor") with a complaint. If something needs specific attention, patients are sent to the specialist in that field. When it comes to headaches and migraines, the specialist is usually an allergist or neurologist.

In either case, it's a mistake to think these people have all the answers; they do not. Yes, they are highly educated in their specific field of treatment, but they are often ignorant of the natural and holistic options and therapies available or any therapy or approach outside their realm of specific expertise. Oftentimes, they dismiss such options as nonsense. This is a shame because there are dozens and dozens of holistic treatment modalities that are proven effective[2] when attempting to overcome the pain, duration, frequency, and prevention of headaches and migraines.

If you find my assertion that it's a mistake to believe doctors have a corner on headache knowledge and answers, I ask you to consider what the World Health Organization (WHO) has to say on the subject. In 2011, the WHO released a report stating, "Headache and migraine disorders are greatly underrated and underreported by health systems and receive too little attention..." and "Lack of knowledge among health care providers is the principal clinical barrier to effective headache (including migraine) management."[3]

MISTAKE #10
Thinking a Migraine is Just a Sinus or Tension Headache

Another mistake of misinformation, due to misunderstanding based in physician diagnosis or product commercials, is mistaking a migraine for a sinus or tension headache. Because most people believe (as noted above) that only certain types of people get migraines, most OTC pain relievers are aimed at treating sinus headaches or tension headaches.

To reiterate, many well-intentioned health care professionals just do not have the training in differentiating headache types or are too focused in their specialty, that they misdiagnose headaches. And because migraines are less common than other types of headaches, they are often only officially diagnosed after treatment has failed for other headache-type diagnoses. Moreover, the public is led to believe by television commercials and print ads that they either have allergy/sinus headaches or tension headaches, because the manufactures of these products also believe only a small percentage of people get migraines.

The truth is that many who complain and visit their primary care physician for chronic headaches are actually suffering from migraines. Tellingly, a look at the active ingredients printed on a box of regular OTC headache pills, and the same brand's "tension" and "migraine" products, reveal all three headache-relieving "products" are identical. And, more importantly, the ingredients are nearly-identical (i.e., aspirin, acetaminophen, caffeine) with an effective migraine prescription drug, minus the barbiturates.

It is a mistake to think you don't have a migraine because advertising and lack of understanding lead you down another thought process. Take migraines seriously because they are among the most debilitating headaches and the ones which need the fastest "onset" response to knock them out. If you have a bad headache and take allergy/sinus or tension headache medicine and the pain does not subside but gets worse, stop taking that medication. It's a mistake to take more of the same medication and hope it will do something different because in these cases, the medicine is not geared to the headache type you are experiencing.

I know it can be difficult to know what to believe. Your trusted healthcare provider diagnoses your headaches and advertisements for headache medicine seems to support that diagnosis. But recall my advice above and the quote from the WHO. Who to believe and what to do? The good news is that later in the book I will tell you how to know what type of headache you are having and offer emergency techniques for reducing the pain in the moment. More importantly, the "Headache Relief Action Plan" works for all headaches. By embracing the plan and implementing the steps into your life, you will no longer have to decide from occurrence to occurrence what headache type you have and what treatment to apply. You will prevent them before they occur!

MISTAKE #11
Avoiding Exercise Because It Makes Headaches Worse

Please don't make the mistake of not exercising because you have headaches. Many people actually use headaches and migraines as an excuse to be lazy, stop exercising, lead a sedentary lifestyle, and eventually give up on life. Please don't allow yourself to fall into this trap, emotionally and physically compelling as it can be.

I want you to know that exercise, regularly getting up and moving your body for a period of time, is essential to health, wellness, and quality of life. Exercise burns calories and stored fat, which contains toxins. It promotes the oxygenation of blood vessels and tissue and the movement of blood and lymph. Exercise reduces stress and burns stress hormones like cortisol which cause headaches. Moving the body reduces muscle tension and "knots" and relieves trigger points that can all lead to tension headache. In short, exercise helps prevent headaches by reducing many of their triggers.

If you get headaches, please exercise. Maybe not while in the midst of a very bad headache, but certainly between headaches or while the chronic ones are at a manageable pain point. Later in the book, I present two of the best exercises for headaches and migraines. By following the "Headache Relief Action Plan," you will be able to exercise more and more over time because the frequency, level, and duration of your headaches will decrease and then disappear.

⊕ MISTAKES OF GIVING UP ⊕

MISTAKE #12
Feeling Disempowered Because Headaches Are Hereditary

It is commonly believed that headaches, especially migraines, are passed on through genetics. In other words, some people believe that headaches run in the family and there is nothing you can do about them. This mistaken thinking has occurred because many who get headaches or migraines have at least one parent and perhaps several relatives who also get headaches.

This really is a problem of the chicken and the egg and of nature versus nurture. Yes, it is true that there are people who have chronic headaches and are part of a family where at least one and often several members also get headaches. Yet, the so-called "genetic" headaches have more to do with the lifestyle of the family than of the genetics. Remember my story about my mother and her MSG-laden seasoning, nitrate-filled hot dogs, and chemical floor cleaners? Well, if several people in my family complained of headaches, they would be diagnosed as "genetically running in our family," when in reality it was the things in our "family lifestyle" externally causing the headaches, not our genetics.

For argument's sake, let's say you have had genetic testing done and it shows you have a "headache gene" in your DNA. This still does not mean you have to get headaches. Think about it. Even in families believed to have "genetic headaches," most of the family members do not get headaches. Why? The study of epigenetics tells us that even when someone has a DNA marker for a specific disease, that genetic "switch" does not have to be turned on; it can be left in the "off position" by lifestyle choices that don't flip the switch on. This is cutting-edge science!

Please don't give up because you think headaches run in your genes and therefore nothing can be done to prevent them. This simply is not the case. In the pages of this book, you will learn how to change your lifestyle, how to make better choices, and how to prevent headaches from retaining their control of your life.

MISTAKE #13
Continuing on a Treatment Plan That's Not Working

Keeping mistake number 12 in mind, it is just as serious a mistake to keep doing the things that are proving unsuccessful in stopping your headaches. If you give a natural remedy the time to work as it should, and it falls short for you or does not seem to help you, then it is a mistake to keep doing it. On the same note, continuing along a plan of medication to mask symptoms of headaches and migraines that is not successful in altering the condition in a positive way and prevent their reoccurrence is also a mistake that you should discontinue.

This book provides dozens and dozens of options for overcoming headaches and migraines. Read the entire book and consider which may work best for you, and in which combinations. Then, give it the best effort you can. If after three months of diligently following the Action Plan, (IF you do it properly), and you are not feeling better or headed in that direction, change course a bit and implement the other options in this book. It's a mistake to continue doing what is not working for you because it's stealing time from your life. Move on to the next one and find the mix of products and therapies and practices that, when combined, do what you need them to. Everyone is different. After all, healing is an art, not a science.

MISTAKE #14
Not Giving Natural Therapies Their Due Time

Why don't people use natural therapies as often as toxic and invasive ones? Because their doctors tell them natural methods are bogus or they seem to work too slowly or not to work at all. I know how it feels to be in constant pain, and have my activities severely restricted. I also had a primary care physician who adamantly dismissed alternative medicine across the board, saying there were no studies showing its effectiveness. He obviously never looked because a simple search on PubMed results in tens of thousands of positive studies showing that alternative methods do work.

I know when you experience an acute headache or suffer from chronic headaches that all you want to do is find immediate relief. Oftentimes, the fastest route to that relief is drugs, shots, and surgeries. But please also believe me when I say from experience that these short-term solutions can have some hefty, long-term consequences.

Natural therapies like herbal remedies, supplements, dietary changes, energy medicine, and manual therapies that gently work the energy lines (meridians), the soft tissue and the skeletal system do work. They work very well, but only when given the time to do their job. Yes, they offer relief but they do so over time. They are gentle and take time to correct the imbalances within the body that cause the headache and migraine. Drugs only cover the symptoms of the imbalances while doing nothing to correct them. Even though they work quickly, drugs and surgeries have side effects.

Please do not give up on natural therapies and solutions; it's a mistake you may later regret. Give them time to do what they do in a natural way. Don't just "try" them for a short period or even a single time, and then say they don't work because they didn't meet your expectations of immediate relief. Instead, change your expectation to echo that of the provider or product and then settle in and give it time to make the lasting changes it's meant to create.

"The Headache Relief Action Plan" presented in this book is powerful and life changing. But first, you have to change your thoughts, actions, and beliefs around headaches and make lifestyle changes. And, you must allow this natural approach time to work after living perhaps decades in pain. It's a mistake to give up on a holistic approach because it takes time and effort and personal commitment.

MISTAKE #15
Believing Nothing Can Be Done About Chronic Headaches

Having been a chronic headache sufferer myself, I know you have been through the mill when it comes to finding relief from the chronic and daily suffering that goes with headaches and migraines. You will recall from the end of Chapter 2 we discussed the need for hope and there is plenty of hope when it comes to most cases of headaches and migraines. This notion of hope is so important to a successful outcome of the "Headache Relief Action Plan" outlined in this book. Believing there are no options left – that you have exhausted all options within the medical profession for headache and migraine relief – is a mistake.

There are so many causes and triggers for headaches and migraines and the symptoms associated with it. The good news is that within the treasure chest of alternative medicine and holistic therapies are hundreds of options that can work for you. Please read this book carefully and find the ones that seem to speak to you and your condition. We are all different and require a unique approach, and a different blend of the means and methods. Despite what the medical establishment tells you, there is no one-size-fits-all approach to headache and migraine. That is why what you have been doing has not worked. If it had, you would not be reading this book. But you are, and hope is found within the options presented herein.

CHAPTER REVIEW

- We all make mistakes when it comes to identifying and dealing with headaches and migraines
- Understanding, learning from, and avoiding these mistakes will begin your journey to a life free from chronic headaches and migraines.
- Save yourself time and pain by avoiding the 15 most common headache mistakes.
- These five mistakes are based in **inaction**:
    - Thinking You Don't Need to See a Doctor About Headaches
    - Waiting Too Long to Address Your Headaches
    - Not Doing Anything Because You Think Migraines Don't Last Long

- Not Taking Action Because Headaches Don't Affect Your Quality of Life
  - Not Taking Personal Control of Your Headaches
- Six mistakes stem from **misinformation**:
  - Only Certain Types of People Get Migraines
  - Thinking People Outgrow Their Headaches
  - Not Acknowledging the Big Role Diet Plays in Headaches and Migraines
  - Thinking Doctors and Medical Specialists Have All the Answers
  - Thinking A Migraine Is Just a Sinus or Tension Headache
  - Avoiding Exercise Because It Makes Headaches Worse
- Four mistakes are rooted in **giving up**:
  - Feeling Disempowered Because You Believe Headaches Are Hereditary
  - Continuing on a Treatment Plan That's Not Working
  - Not Giving Natural Therapies Their Due Time
  - Believing Nothing Can Be Done About Chronic Headaches
- Understanding and avoiding these mistakes will greatly improve your success with the Headache Relief Action Plan.

CHAPTER 5

HOW FOOD IMPACTS HEADACHE AND MIGRAINE

Do you wake up in the morning tired, with only enough time to devour a plain bagel and cup of coffee? For lunch, do you settle for a quick cold cuts sandwich and a soft drink? For dinner, do you enjoy a nice Italian meal complete with red wine, coffee and dessert? If you answered yes to one or all of these questions and suffer chronic headaches, then food definitely is a trigger for you, as it is for millions of other chronic headache sufferers.

One of the most difficult things people struggle with is diet and food choices, which directly impact headaches. In this chapter, we'll discuss how your food choices can exponentially impact the frequency, level and duration of headaches and migraines.

In the previous chapter, we learned how allergies or sensitivities to chemicals play a major role in headaches. Low blood sugar and high levels of fat in the blood are also notorious headache triggers; as are low levels of serotonin, the chemical tyramine, nightshades (also known as the Solanaceae, a family of flowering plants), dairy, and more. Let's take a broad look at the list of foods that are known triggers of headaches and migraines.

- **Animal Milk Products:** Milk, Cream, Ice Cream, Cheese, Cottage Cheese, Yogurt
- **Hydrogenated Oils:** Non-Dairy Creamer, Crackers, Cookies, Chips, Snack Bars
- **Nitrates**: Hot Dogs, Cold Cuts, Pepperoni, Sausage, Bacon, Liverwurst
- **Processed Sugars:** Candy, Soda, Bread, Bottled Fruit Juice, Cookies, Snack Bars
- **Nightshades:** White Potatoes, Eggplants, Sweet and Hot Peppers, Tomatoes, Tomatillos, Tamarios, Pepinos, Pimentos, Goji Berries, Ground Cherries, Cape Gooseberries, Garden Huckleberries and Paprika
- **Fast Foods:** French Fries, Onion Rings, Loaded Baked Potatoes, Fatty Burgers, Mexican Food, Pizza, Calzones, Strombolis
- **Caffeine:** Coffee, Black Tea, Soda, Chocolate
- **Saturated Fats:** Marbleized Beef, Chuck Ground Beef, Deep Fried Foods, Chicken Skin
- **Processed White Foods:** Flour, Bread, Pasta, Sugar, Artificial Sweeteners

Let's now look at how these areas affect the body and trigger headaches.

CHRONIC LOW-GRADE INFLAMMATION

Food is also a critical piece of the puzzle when it comes to controlling inflammation and headache triggers. Inflammation is the body's way of telling you something is wrong and in need of change. Most people live with chronic low-grade inflammation. Inflammation, then, is both a sign and a symptom of pain, especially headaches and migraines.

The amount of inflammation in your body varies and is dependent on a number of factors -- your activity level, the amount of sleep you get, the degree of stress in your life, and yes... even the food you eat. What you have to realize is that these factors are cumulative; they build up over time. And the more that any or all of these factors become out of control, your risk for disease increases.

Nightshades are particularly troublesome for those who suffer with headaches and migraines. These foods can cause calcification, bone spurs, and inflammation. These side effects are deleterious to those suffering with headaches and migraines. In cases of people who are sensitive or allergic to nightshades, they can cause nerve damage, muscle tremors, and impede digestion.

Milk-based products are also troublesome for those suffering with headaches and migraines. They are often high in cholesterol and saturated fat, and can contribute to obesity and cause mucus for form, which cause headaches. Moreover, products like milk, yogurt, ice cream, cheese, cottage cheese, and various sauces can contribute to an increase in phlegm-rheum. Phlegm-rheum is a classification of thick, sticky fluids in the body that include mucus. These thick and sticky fluids put pressure on the sinuses and are a perfect environment for bacteria and increased inflammation and pain. One of the things you will learn about in the book is how to dry the body of such sticky fluids to improve circulation, reduce swelling and inflammation, and also decrease pain.

The sweetener known as high fructose corn syrup (HFCS) has been identified as the main culprit in the rise of youth obesity in the United States. As we discussed, obesity is one of the key risks for headaches and migraines. High fructose corn syrup is corn syrup that has undergone enzymatic processing to convert its glucose into fructose. This fructose has then been mixed with regular corn syrup, which is 100% glucose, and the result is a sweet liquid known as high fructose.

This liquid is the sweetener found in just about every cold beverage in your local convenience store, including iced tea, sodas. and energy drinks. Not only that, but it is also found in so-called healthy foods like tomato soup and yogurt, and less healthful items such as salad dressings and cookies. The FDA did a 30-year study and found a correlation between HFCS and obesity, stating that it is worse for your health than plain sugar, which also is not good for those with chronic headaches and migraine.

ALCOHOL AND CAFFEINE

Alcohol has been causing headaches since the first drink was poured. Aside from your basic hangover resulting from over-consumption of this adult beverage, even small amounts of alcohol can trigger headaches in a number of ways. For starters, alcohol is a vasodilator, which means it not only contributes to rebound headaches but also hinders the liver's ability to metabolize carbohydrates. When carbohydrates are not properly broken down or burned off through exercise, your body changes their excess to glucose, which raises blood sugar levels, and activates the release of insulin. If there is too much alcohol in the bloodstream, too much insulin will be released and cause blood sugar levels to fall too low, and a hypoglycemic headache will result. What's more, even when alcohol is eliminated from the body through sweating, urine, and feces, it leaves behind a fat byproduct that not only causes toxicity but also causes blood fat levels to rise. Both of these can cause headaches. For chronic headache sufferers, it is best to either abstain from alcohol completely or limit intake to only a few times per year.

Among the most notorious chemicals in our everyday diet that induces headaches is caffeine. Coffee, black or green tea, most soft drinks, cocoa and many over-the-counter medications (e.g., Excedrin, cough syrups) are the main culprits in serving copious amounts of caffeine to the populous. The sheer amount of this legally addictive stimulant Americans consume each year in the form of coffee itself is ridiculous—in excess of 10 pounds per person!

Like most food sensitivities, caffeine can trigger headaches in a number of ways, including toxic pesticides and other chemicals used in growing coffee. Coffee's natural acids and oils and stimulant property triggers the rebound headache effect. In addition, like alcohol, caffeine is a natural diuretic and leads to dehydration. It also causes breathing difficulties and insomnia, stress and anxiety, imbalances in blood sugar and cholesterol levels, dilation and constriction of blood vessels, and depletion of vitamins and minerals such as potassium, magnesium, essential B vitamins, thiamine and vitamin C. Each one of these side effects by itself is a known headache trigger. Think of how the united effect of caffeine's effects can wreak havoc on the body's ability to maintain homeostasis, and their impact on manifesting any combination of "mixed" headaches (migraine, tension type, toxic, rebound, sensitivity).

If you think you're safe drinking decaffeinated coffee, think again. Not only do most decaffeinated brands still contain 7% caffeine, but methylene chloride, the main chemical used in the decaffeination process, is toxic to the body. If you simply love coffee so much that you just can't live without it, decaf is your best bet as long as it has been decaffeinated using what is known as the Swiss water process, and the beans themselves are certified organic.

BLOOD SUGAR AND BLOOD FAT

Low blood sugar, high blood sugar, and high blood fat have been proven in hundreds of clinical studies to trigger headaches (among a host of other ailments and diseases). Since rises and decreases in levels of blood sugar and fat are caused by our dietary *choices*, they are avoidable and their resultant headaches can also be avoided. Among the culprits of increased blood sugars and fats are a diet made up of mainly refined sugar (sucrose), animal and hydrogenated fats, simple carbohydrates, caffeinated and alcoholic beverages, dehydration, and the skipping of meals.

Sugar in the body is not always bad and it is actually necessary, as long as the sugar is the right kind. You see, the human body is biologically set up for the effective breakdown and use of *fructose*, or the natural sugar found in fruits and vegetables. During the digestive process, the body breaks fructose down and turns it into glucose or blood sugar, our primary source of energy. An abundance of *glucose* also triggers the release of insulin, which not only stabilizes blood sugar levels but also metabolizes fat in the body.

Problems arise for the chronic headache sufferer when *sucrose*, or refined sugar, enters the bloodstream. While fructose is nature's natural sugar and glucose is the body's broken down version for energy use, sucrose is an unnatural hybrid of the two natural forms of sugar and is extremely difficult for the body to metabolize. Overconsumption of sucrose leads to toxic buildup in the blood stream and causes blood sugar levels to rise and then fall from the release of too much insulin, thus creating both toxic and rebound headaches.

There is a direct correlation between sugar levels in the body and blood fat levels, and both can cause headaches independent of the other. The best way to prevent headaches brought on as a result of "bad" blood sugars levels and high levels of cholesterol and triglycerides in the blood stream is a diet rich in whole grains, complex carbohydrates, vegetables, fruits, grains, protein foods, water, and the abstinence of beverages high in caffeine and alcohol content.

SEROTONIN AND TYRAMINE

One of the main chemical triggers of migraine headaches is a low level of serotonin in the body. Serotonin in a monoamine neurotransmitter that carries information from nerve ends to different parts of the body, where it is detected by special receptors and causes a wide range of reactions.

Serotonin also plays the lead role in controlling depression, anxiety, eating and sleeping patterns, inhibiting pain, and preventing blood vessels from dilating too much. When serotonin levels are low, blood vessels dilate causing headaches; sleep is also disrupted, resulting in headaches; depression sets in causing inactivity and eating disorders, which cause headaches; and, pain is able to move easily and powerfully among the nerve endings.

Numerous scientific studies and clinical trials have shown a clear relationship between low levels of serotonin and headaches. In one such study, when injected with a drug that depletes serotonin, test subjects got headaches. Likewise, when they were injected with serotonin, the headache went away.[1]

There are a number of things that cause serotonin levels to drop, including a lack of vitamin B6 and tryptophan and ingestion of high levels of tyramine. All of these are directly linked to diet. Essential B vitamins and tryptophan are found in many fruits, vegetables, grains and legumes, and a lack of essential vitamins and minerals in the body reflects poor eating habits. Caffeine is also known to deplete vitamin B.

Tyramine is a vasoactive amino acid found in foods and is thought to dilate blood vessels. Foods that contain tyramine may cause headaches in migraine sufferers by facilitating a chain reaction that results in selective cerebral vasoconstriction (the most common cause of headache pain) followed by rebound dilation of the cranial vessels. This sequence is implicated in migraine headache.

Maintaining proper elevated levels of serotonin is vital for chronic headache sufferers in general, and for migraine sufferers in particular. This is as easy (or as difficult) as eating a diet high in complex carbohydrates, rich in legumes, seeds and grains, moderate in protein, and low in tyramine-containing foods. These foods elevate tryptophan levels in the body, which are essential for the production of serotonin.

pH IMBALANCES

You know how acidic fruits like lemons, can "eat" the enamel off your teeth and how acids can corrode a battery casing? Well, your body can become overly acidic, too, when the natural pH or ratio of acid to base (alkaline) is off kilter.

The initials pH refer to the scientific term "potential hydrogen." This is the concentration of hydrogen ions in the body. The pH scale has a range of 0-14, with the sweet spot for human blood being around 7.35. As the numbers increase, the body becomes more alkaline; however, as the numbers decrease, the body becomes more acidic. Being in a constant or chronic acidic state is not only unhealthy, it is damaging to the body.

The human body was not designed to withstand chronic acidic states. When the body is off-balance long enough, and out of its natural state of homeostasis, it starts to break down. Signs and symptoms of an excessively acidic body can be seen and/or felt externally with the onset of headaches, body pain, and skin rashes. In the acidic range, the immune system is compromised, leading to easily contracted sinus infections, allergies, and cold and flu, placing you at risk for progressing autoimmune diseases, headaches, and migraines. Moreover, an acidic interior environment can lead to muscle contractions that restrict the free flow of blood and inhibit the exchange of nutrients and waste products from muscle cells. This can cause soreness, cramping, fatigue, degenerative cellular diseases, and even cellular death.

Pain is correlated with pH imbalance and a chronic acid state within the body. Thankfully, you don't have to worry about this when your body is kept within the alkaline range of 7.0-7.4. In fact, while in this range it is impossible for disease to sustain itself because the immune system is strong and there is no longer an acidic environment necessary for diseases, like cancer, gout, headaches, and migraines. This chart will help you see how the foods you eat and the beverages you drink contribute to an unhealthy internal environment.

	0	Battery Acid
	1	Stomach Acid
	2	Lemon Juice, Vinegar
Acid	3	Orange Juice, Soda
	4	Tomato Juice, Beer
	5	Black Coffee
	6	Saliva, Cow's Milk
Neutral	7	Pure Water
	8	Sea Water
	9	Baking Soda
	10	Antacid
Alkaline	11	Ammonia
	12	Soapy Water
	13	Bleach, Oven Cleaner
	14	Drain Cleaner

pH Balance Chart

An imbalanced pH or acid/alkaline interior environment is one of the hidden causes of headaches and migraines and one of the states that make symptoms worse. How does the body become too acidic and thus unhealthy, placing you at risk for negative health symptoms, such as those associated with headaches and migraines? Well, stress is a big one. Stress, or the effects of being in the "fight or flight" response for too long a period of time releases stress hormones into the body, flooding the blood stream with protective chemicals. These chemicals, like cortisol, were necessary during the time of our great ancestors who had to run for their lives from wild beasts or head hunting tribes. These days, the stress response happens from different types of stressors, like emotional upset, physically demanding work, and overwhelming psychological issues that we deal with at home and at work. There are too many of these happening throughout the day in our modern lives. It is no wonder we are under chronic states of stress, are not well, and are in constant acidic states. Dealing with stress is huge when it comes to reducing the symptoms of headaches and migraines. In Chapter 16, I will show you how to do it, naturally.

Our modern diet is also a huge contributor to our chronic, acidic interior environment. When food reaches your digestive tract, it is broken down and either leaves an alkaline or an acidic residue behind. If one eats foods that are organic, whole, and fresh, and drinks plenty of pure water, the body can easily maintain an alkaline state. However, consuming sugar, refined grains, preservatives, pesticides, dairy products such as cow's milk, cheese, yogurt and ice cream, red meat, chocolate, coffee, soda, and alcohol turns the body acidic. One of the main culprits of poor diet is inflammation, which is also the main symptom of headache and migraine and pain.

As mentioned earlier, pH is a measure of the potential hydrogen or residue a food leaves behind, and is either alkaline or acidic. And this is not directly related to the acidic nature of a food before it is digested. Lemons, for example, are highly acidic. If you squeeze the juice of a lemon on an open wound, it will burn. However, when ingested and digested, lemon is very alkalizing for the body and lemon juice can help reduce acidic levels. A diet that is low in acidic foods and packed full of nutrient-dense alkalizing foods will make you healthier while also reducing the symptoms of headaches and migraines. This diet is explained later in the book.

If you have headaches and migraines, suffer symptoms like pain and stiffness, and have a predisposition to infection, it is likely that an imbalanced pH is present in your body. To be sure, you can purchase pH testing strips or rolls in your local drug store. These are thin paper items that gauge your pH level when dipped into your saliva or urine stream first thing in the morning before you eat or drink anything. What your end goal should be is to be in either the alkaline range (7.0-7.4) or moving toward it.

Natural methods of reducing the acidic environment in your body in favor of alkalizing it will be shared in the chapters dealing with diet, supplements, and mind-body techniques. In the meantime, please control this unhealthy, interior environment by avoiding or severely restricting the foods mentioned in this chapter.

In Chapter 9, I present a pro-alkaline and anti-inflammatory diet for headache prevention. It is important to view food in terms of how it affects the body. It can make it stronger or weaker – that is, every cell, organ, tissue, bone, tendon, muscle, and fluid. All of these affect headaches and migraines, so a diet that is nutrient dense, anti-inflammatory, and free of chemical pesticides, while also providing a boost to blood flow and the feel-good hormones, is what you want to embrace. I will tell you the how's and why's and show you how to put it into place.

CHAPTER REVIEW

- Food can cause pain and inflammation – you have the power to improve your headache and migraine symptoms through diet.

- Avoid fatty, sugary, and processed foods to stave off pain and inflammation.

- Avoid alcohol and caffeine to help stabilize your neurological and vascular systems.

- Monitor your internal pH to keep your body from harboring an acidic environment – a step that is critical to improving pain from inflammation.

- Your diet is an important part of the solution to achieving a life free from chronic headaches and migraines.

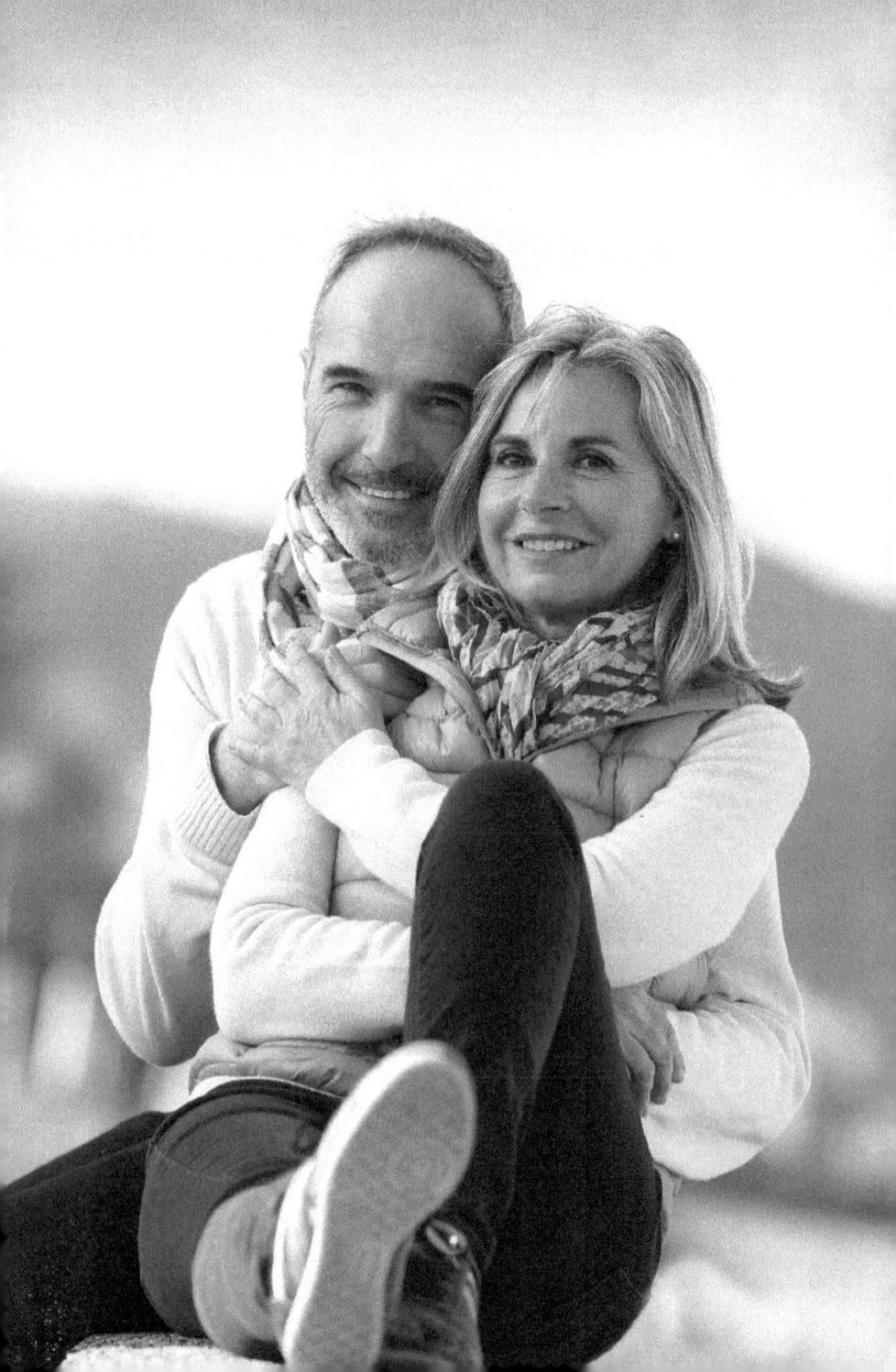

CHAPTER 6

HOW STRESS AND EMOTIONS AFFECT HEADACHES

The content of your mind and the state of your emotions play a vital role in both wellness and illness. Emotions are natural and play an important part in our lives. However, in excess or stagnation, emotions can be damaging to the body. Many who suffer chronic headaches and migraines also suffer from chronic stress, mental and emotional fatigue, an inability to make decisions, and depression. Often times these emotional states are a result of experiencing headaches or being diagnosed with migraines. These states of being cause pain and inflammation that worsen and lead to feelings of hopelessness.

Please believe me when I tell you *this doesn't need not to be the case!* Something more can be done, and, in many cases a lot more can be done to help you. Reading this chapter will help tremendously because it puts your headaches and their symptoms in context with your thoughts and feelings. Once you come to see how mind and emotions, often directed by stress, affect you for better or worse, you will be able to embrace more fully the mind-body techniques explored later in the book. These will be of tremendous help to you in overcoming the frequency, severity, and duration of your headaches.

Your mind and emotions play key roles in how you experience your headaches and migraines and in the potential outcome of your success when implementing "The Headache Relief Action Plan." Understanding this link is a key component of finding relief and deriving a better quality of life. Let's look at why this is the case.

THE MIND-BODY CONNECTION

Stress is one of the leading causes of illness in the United States, and it is one of the main triggers of headaches. The effects of stress include a racing mind, obsessive thoughts, unending worry, muscle tension and spasm, poor or too great an appetite, digestive disorders, constipation, insomnia, poor blood flow, belabored breathing, neck and shoulder tension, and the possible onset or continuation of bad habits such as dependence on alcohol, drugs, pain killers, food, and caffeine. Any one of these things by itself can trigger any number of different types of headaches. But when these antagonistic forces are combined (as they generally are when triggered by stress), the headache problem can become chronic and insufferable.

Stress erodes your health and undermines your quality of life. It is a psychosomatic response to what is happening around you. Put another way, stress is a physical manifestation in the body of what the mind perceives and struggles with.

The term *psychosomatic* was once used by psychologists to identify pain or illnesses that were assumed to be "all in the mind" of the patient, and, therefore, "not real." This outlook is dated and false. The seed of the physical condition *is* in the thoughts and emotions of the person affected by them. However, these symptoms are not "imaginary"; they are felt in the body in very real ways. Indeed, they exist in very real forms, such as inflammation, swelling, spasms, trigger points, pain, anxiety, stress, and depression. This "pain body," as Eckhart Tolle refers to it, is the leading cause of chronic pain, especially joint pain, muscle pain, fibromyalgia, migraine, and chronic headaches. Dr. John Sarno refers to the phenomenon as Tension Myositis Syndrome (TMS), which is discussed later in the book.

The answer to the puzzle of how the mind affects the body and the body affects the mind may well be found within the mind itself and the hold it has over your thoughts, emotions and the quality of your physical body. When the mind (psycho) and the body (soma) come together in adverse ways to manifest pain, inflammation, rashes, muscle spasms…it is called psychosomatic illness. This term is just a technical way of saying there is a direct connection and relationship between your mind and your body. The mind-body (psychosomatic) connection is a real, two-way street. Your mind affects your body and your body affects your mind. How?

Well, when you think your condition is bad and that nothing can be done, you release stress hormones that negatively affect your health over time and your feelings of well-being in the moment. These then create negative cycles of stress and anxiety that can lead to depression. These emotions decrease your energy, slow your breathing, decrease your blood flow, and make you unmotivated to get up and move. This causes muscle tightness, weight gain, loss of range of motion, inflammation, and pain.

You see, it is interrelated. When your body feels in pain or cannot do what you ask of it, this affects your mind and emotions.

When your mind and emotions are too negative, you begin to feel worse, experience more pain, and stop doing things you used to enjoy. This causes more of the symptoms that make your condition feel worse and deteriorate it faster. Stress plays a large role in this.

THE STRESS RESPONSE

It all starts with stress derived from worry about your headache condition, the loss of activity and joy in your life, and how you'll fare in the years to come. Stress and worry are major components of how you perceive your pain and headache condition, and, also play a part in how your headaches and migraines begin and develop. As stated in the introduction, not everyone experiences headaches in the same way and not all headaches are the same.

You are not alone in this physical manifestation of pain based in thoughts and beliefs; it is part of the human condition and how we are programmed. Stress is one of the leading causes of illness in the United States. Nearly 66% of all signs and symptoms presented in doctors' offices in the U.S. are stress induced. And the symptoms most associated with headaches are known to be aggravated, and often severely increased by stress.

What happens when you are under stress – real or perceived – is that your body moves through a *stress response*. Through the physiological mechanism of stress, your muscles tighten, which inhibits circulation and constricts blood vessels, causing stiffness, trigger points, inflammation, and limited range of motion and pain. The hypertonic (painfully tight) muscles place a compressive load on the vertebra, especially those of the neck (cervical) and the trigger points slow the flow of blood and the exchange of blood, oxygen, and nutrients.

The effects of stress include nail biting, anxiety, a racing mind, obsessive thoughts, compulsive behavior, unending worry, muscle tension and spasm, poor appetite, overeating, digestive disorders, constipation, insomnia, poor blood flow, belabored breathing, neck pain, shoulder tension and the possible onset or continuation of bad habits such as dependence on alcohol, drugs, painkillers, food and caffeine. All of these responses to stress are headache triggers by themselves. When combined, they become the perfect storm for long-lasting, acute migraine and chronic headache conditions.

THE NASTY CYCLE

While all of the above reactions to stress are normal, they are not necessary or healthy to maintain. In fact, when left unchecked, stress actually triggers a cycle of worry about those symptoms, which then makes your headaches and their symptoms worse. Round and round it goes until stress, anxiety, and depression become your dominant mental framework and emotional set point. This can make you feel like your condition is helpless, that nothing can be done to improve it, and that you will live an unhappy, severely hampered life.

Again, these mental and emotional states have a negative impact on the nervous system and take a toll on the body. Without adequate blood flow, the cells in your body become slightly oxygen deprived. Toxins and waste aren't cleaned out and removed as efficiently as they should be, and this build up creates or reactivates trigger points in certain parts of your body. These knots are often painful to the touch, and, in some cases, cause muscles to spasm or "lock-up," which can compress your arthritic joints, causing even greater pain, inflammation, restricted range of motion, stress, frustration, and depression.

Without fresh blood supplying oxygen and nutrients, it is nearly impossible to heal. Stress also alters your breathing. Typically, when you are anxious or upset, your breath becomes shallow, reducing oxygen flow to the whole body. Oxygen and nutrients don't circulate at optimum levels, which again contribute to the buildup of toxins. Stress also can release hormones, such as adrenaline and cortisol, which can trigger chronic tension and systemic low grade inflammation. Increased levels of cortisol cause fat to accumulate across your midsection and affects heart health and increases your chances of becoming overweight. Without adequate blood flow to remove these hormones from the body, they can linger longer than usual and create more damage.

The effect of such prolonged or recurring stress is that the autonomic nervous system is kept from balancing, which can lead to problems with the gastrointestinal tract, the digestive system, the respiratory system, and the neuroendocrine system. When coupled with headaches and migraines, stress can also lead to depression, which can lock in an almost permanent, negative mental and emotional state that can be hard to overcome.

Depression affects more than 20 million Americans and represents a serious mental health problem. Depression is believed to have a genetic basis, and change the chemical composition of the brain, where symptoms like loss of energy, fatigue, and prolonged feelings of deep sadness, loss of interest in things, and even thoughts of suicide stay front and center for an extended period.

Many folks treat depression with psychotherapy or prescription antidepressant drugs. Although many experts think a combination of these two are effective, no scientific evidence supports this supposition. In reality, research shows that simple, natural measures like more sleep, exercise, supplementation, diet and efforts at *sustaining a positive attitude work better to combat depression than medication.*

WHAT YOU THINK BECOMES YOUR REALITY

A lot has been written and lectured about the Law of Attraction. The works of Abraham-Hicks, Wayne Dyer, Deepak Chopra, and Eckhart Tolle have given people a better understanding of the way in which our minds not only affect but create our perceptions and our lives. If perception is reality, then what you think (the content of your mind) forms your belief system. Your belief system affects how you then see the world and how you in turn respond to it. This includes your perception of headaches and how they do and will affect you.

The mind is inextricably connected to the body. If you want to be healthy and happy instead of in pain and feeling sick, you have to readjust your attitude toward health. Healthy people are happy people. And shifting your attitude from "nothing helps" to "I can make better choices" is often the key step that offers optimal wellness and emotional fulfillment. Health and happiness represent a frame of mind that influences your choices. Making better lifestyle choices leads to wellness and a better quality of life.

It is absolutely necessary and vital that you work toward thinking positively about yourself, your life, and your headache condition. Let your emotions be your guide in self-regulating stress and the mind-body cycle. When you feel bad, reframe your mind with the techniques taught in Section II. Searching for and finding the positive in all aspects of life will attract more positive thoughts and feelings. These will decrease the stress and anxiety of headaches, help stave off depression, and keep you as active as you can be. This will help you better follow the program outlined in Section III and swipe away the negative impact that chronic headaches and migraines have on your life.

Chapters 16 and 17 present dozens of natural and proven methods and strategies for combating the emotional distress and stress of chronic headaches, and also offers treatment methods and self-help modalities for overcoming headaches. Take some time to review Section I, and then begin Section II with a fresh mind and invigorated spirit.

CHAPTER REVIEW

- Don't let your pain be worsened by stress and mental and emotional fatigue.
- Understand your mind and body are intricately interconnected; negative emotions increase your pain and multiply your physical symptoms.
- By simply readjusting your attitude and outlook toward your health and headache conditions using positivity, you can experience fewer headache days, and shorter and less intense headaches.
- Let your emotions be your guide in self-regulating stress and the mind-body cycle.
- Read Chapter 9 for techniques on how to reframe your mind toward better health.

CHAPTER 7

THE THREE HIDDEN IMBALANCES THAT CAUSE HEADACHES

The secret of overcoming headaches and migraines is to understand where they begin. The Headaches Relief Action Plan is built on correcting the three *hidden imbalances* that derail your health and actually cause pain, illness, and disease, including headaches and migraines. These hidden imbalances are the beginnings — or root causes — that must be understood before you can truly understand and believe in the action plan for relieving them. You can then make changes in your lifestyle that stop perpetuating the three hidden causes and instead create an internal homeostatic balance wherein it is difficult for the headache triggers to take hold, and, control your life.

The causes of headaches are quite vast, and, yet, they all have something in common: they are based on a combination of one of three types or categories of imbalance. These imbalance categories are known as **Excesses** (too much of something), **Deficiencies** (too little of something) and **Stagnation** (things moving too slowly). For short, I will refer to this concept simply as EDS (excess/deficiency/stagnation). The concept of excesses, stagnation, and deficiency has its roots in Chinese medicine and how it views the pulse and organ systems. I, personally, apply the concept more broadly and use it to inform my work and as a basis of the "Headache Relief Action Plan" (and also use it in the "Arthritis Relief Action Plan," featured in my book *Arthritis Reversed*). To understand what is meant by these terms, let's first consider *homeostasis* – the body's natural state of balance.

THE BASELINE OF HEALTH

Homeostasis is the body's baseline of health and well-being. It is the state where you feel good and centered. It is a state of being wherein you are neither too stressed, too tired nor too excited. You are in a state where your digestion is working properly, your body is absorbing proper amounts of nutrients and oxygen, and you are efficiently expelling toxins through the skin, lungs, urine, and intestines. Your sleep and wake cycle is set, you work and exercise, and you have a balanced home-work-social life. Things are good.

But life often gets in the way and we don't feel as good anymore. Poor health, pain, and disease are all felt in a body that it is off balance, and no longer functioning at homeostasis. This happens when you experience or engage in excesses (e.g., too much alcohol, exercise or work), deficiencies (e.g., not enough sleep or too little exercise) or stagnations (e.g., muscle spasms or constipation).

People suffer needlessly every day because they and their healthcare practitioners operate from a disease-based model of health. "Mr. Smith, you have headache pain, so we will treat the pain of the headache with this medication." This approach obviously does not work because millions of people still suffer from the pain of headaches. It fails to get at the root cause of what is triggering the headaches in the first place, which are the things that cause imbalances in your body and mind.

HEADACHES AND THE EDS PUZZLE

I propose you begin to consider your overall health — your headache condition and its symptoms in particular — as examples of imbalances. Below, you will learn more about the specifics of the three hidden EDS imbalances. Apply the concept to your life and see where and when and how these may be the root cause of what triggers your headaches and migraines. The "Headache Relief Action Plan" accounts for these, generally and specifically, so the answer to "What do I do with this information?" will be made clear later in the book.

The three terms that comprise EDS revolve around the idea that to reduce the pain level, duration, and frequency of your headaches, and to live as symptom-free as possible, you need to maintain a balance within and between your body, mind and diet. In other words, you need to make changes to your lifestyle. It's important to avoid too much (i.e., excess) of anything that causes your condition or symptoms to get worse, or too little (i.e., deficiency) of something to prevent it from getting better. Let's now take a look at this concept of "three hidden causes" as it is associated with the connection between your body, mind, and diet (i.e., your lifestyle) and the headaches and migraine you suffer.

Headaches Excesses

Too much of a bad thing and too much of a good thing create imbalances in the body that have consequences. This is certainly true when it comes to headaches. When we consider how headaches develop, we will see it begins with chemical and neurological changes in the body that cause pain.

This is often the result of too much (or an *excess* of) imbalanced physical activity. As stated earlier in the book, exercise is needed to help reduce headache triggers. However, too much of rigorous forms like power lifting, long-distance running, and high-impact aerobics can lead to muscle strain and spasm, tendon strain, a raise in blood pressure, and pain in the spine that affects the nerves. Jarring movements from running and jumping and the stress and strain from lifting heaving weights, along with the lactic acid that results from "too much, too fast" can cause a host of excess imbalances that trigger headaches.

A diet that is in excess of artificial sweeteners, nitrates, nightshade vegetables and fruits, alcohol and caffeine is also detrimental to those prone to chronic headaches or migraines. What we consume in the form of food and beverages are among the most prevalent headache and migraine triggers. The list of specific "trigger foods" is presented later in the book, but their excessive consumption leads to chemical changes in the body that directly cause headaches and migraines.

Emotions (how we think and feel about things), as we learned in the previous chapter, play a big role in your headache experiences. First, some have a mindset for success that leads them to push, push, push to get things done; to run the extra mile; to eat while working and then to forgo rest and relaxation. This Type-A personality can actually contribute to getting both forms of headaches. The excessive pushing behavior wears down the body and triggers headaches by increasing stress hormones and reducing sleep.

The next part is the preponderance (excess) of low-vibration emotions that comes once you have been diagnosed with headaches. Wallowing in sorrow for too long, chronically feeling that nothing can be, and complaining to everyone are all ways in which an excess of negative emotion can derail progress. Headaches can feel worse than they are and can increase in pain and duration when you embrace a life excessively ripe with negative thoughts, feelings, and emotions.

The good news is that all of the excess hidden triggers are dealt with in the "Headache Relief Action Plan."

Headaches Deficiencies

When it comes to headaches, deficiencies play a role in cause and effect. If you have a diet that lacks the appropriate amount of whole, fresh and organic fruits and vegetables, you are depriving your body of the nutrients necessary for growth and strength. Blood, bone, muscle and tendon health are so important for preventing headaches and reducing their frequency. The body needs nutrition to be healthy and a body deficient in foods that go bad or rot (as opposed to processed, packaged foods) develops an imbalance.

Drinking too little water is also an issue because water keeps the tissues moist, the joints lubricated, and the tendons and muscles supple. Dehydration does not allow the body to remove enough of the impurities and toxins that stress it. When these are left to recycle in the body, they can cause pain, inflammation and what Chinese medicine refers to as "blood stagnation," making headaches worse.

Exercise, like diet, is a two-edge sword. As mentioned above, too much can cause headaches but too little can also cause headaches because the body needs exercise to invigorate the blood, circulation, maintain and improve cardiovascular health, and oxygenate the body.

If you do not focus on positive outcomes and take ownership of your headaches, you will not be able to make powerful strides toward slowing their frequency and reducing their duration and pain. Too little stake in your own health and making the necessary lifestyle changes is one of the detrimental, downward spirals people get into once they are diagnosed with chronic headaches and migraines. Please don't allow yourself to be among them.

Headaches Stagnations

When it comes to headaches there needs to be a "moving along" of the stagnations that trigger them. Generally speaking, these are experienced as tight, inflexible muscles in spasm that compress the spinal vertebra and cause pressure on the nerves (especially the trigeminal nerve). Muscle spasms cause trigger points, which lock toxins within the muscle tissue, preventing fresh blood and oxygen to move freely in them, which causes stiffness, localized pain, and referred pain in the head. When the body is in one place too long, like prolonged sitting or lying, it is stagnating in place. This is unhealthy, especially for headaches, which require a body that is regularly moving to prevent symptoms.

Remaining in a holding pattern in terms of diet and nutrition is also a form of stagnation. It means you have not made up your mind and committed to eating the right kinds of foods that help prevent headaches and passing on the foods that trigger them. It also means taking the supplementation necessary to help effect positive change. One of the key symptoms of a poor diet is constipation—a stagnation of waste product in the intestines that trigger migraines through toxic re-assimilation into the blood.

Don't stagnate when it comes to diet and supplementation. Make a change, even if it is a small change each week.

Your mind and emotions can also stagnate or control you through their focus on the negative. Stress and anxiety make it hard to make decisions because you are worried about an outcome or afraid to begin a plan of change. Indecision is in fact a form of mental stagnation that causes, according to the theories of traditional Chinese medicine (TCM), "Liver Qi Stagnation," which in turn causes "Liver Fire" (a heating of the liver), which then causes "liver blood" to rise to the head, resulting in a red face and headaches on the top or vertex of the head.

When you don't change your view on the subject of headaches, your mind and emotions stagnate in the realm of the negative. This can create a negative world view and halt (stagnate) change. Again, as with nutrition, you can make small daily changes in how you view your condition and can then create changes in behavior (and in your condition) over time. This can be hard at times, but it is vitally necessary.

Look at these two charts. The first, shows how the "Three Hidden Causes" are likely the "root" of your condition, and how they affect it. The second shows how the symptoms you experience are also related to excesses, deficiencies and stagnations.

RESTORING BALANCE IS THE KEY

It would be a mistake to assume that only one of these three causes is the root of any health condition, especially a condition as complex as chronic headaches and migraines. In fact, it is usually a combination of all three EDSs that make a simple problem become chronic and seemingly complex. The first "cause" of an issue could be singular (i.e., an excess), but when not approached with the wellness model of health (i.e., restoring balance), it becomes multi-faceted.

The way to reduce the frequency, duration, and pain of your headaches and migraines is to consider them and your daily thoughts, beliefs, and actions (i.e., lifestyle) from this three-part "hidden cause" perspective. If you can categorize where you are in excess, you can then make changes toward decrease and balance. If you are able to list areas of deficiency, you can then take steps to improve them. Where you find stagnations, you can look for ways to "move them along."

Returning the body to homeostasis – natural wellness balance – can be difficult and challenging. You may have been polluting your body with toxins in foods, beverages, and air and aggravating it with stress, tension, insufficient sleep, and poor lifestyle choices for quite some time.

In order to re-establish natural wellness balance, the many toxins and stressors that tax the body must be removed or, in the case of psychosomatic triggers, dealt with in new ways. This includes reducing food triggers, correcting musculoskeletal triggers, regulating biological functions, reducing the effects of stress and anxiety, keeping the body in a perpetual state of proper hydration, and engaging in regular exercise. Don't worry, it may sound daunting but the "Headache Relief Action Plan" presented later in this book is structured around ways to do just that.

A DANGEROUS CYCLE

I hope you will find it easy to understand how these three EDS concepts – too much, too little and too slow – can trigger, contribute to, and aggravate headaches and migraines. It is important to know that the EDSs happen at the same time. Consuming too much alcohol can mean you are consuming too little water. Too much fast food generally means too little leafy green veggies. Too little exercise means you are sitting for too long. Too much stress generally presents with little meditation or sleep. And the cycle of relationships continues in a spiral of its own momentum. It is a dangerous and self-reinforcing cycle that must be broken for the successful prevention of chronic headaches and migraines.

To change that cycle, you will need to make lifestyle changes and embrace methods of treatment that may seem out of the ordinary to you at this time. The goal is to restore balance in your life, body, thoughts, emotions, and diet to create a positive change that can add great joy and years of quality to your life.

The "Headache Relief Action Plan" entails lifestyle changes. Making such changes is the only way to correct imbalances and move toward an optimal state of health. In Section II, we'll look at the various modalities, diets, and methods proven effective in reducing and preventing headaches and migraines.

CHAPTER REVIEW

- The secret to overcoming headaches lies in understanding where they begin.
- Three hidden imbalances derail your health and cause pain, illness, and disease.
- Despite multiple types of headaches and their myriad of causes, all are triggered by a combination of three types of imbalance or hidden causes.
- Restoring balance of Excesses, Deficiencies, and Stagnations is key to reversing headaches.
- You can prevent headaches by correcting those imbalances and fully embracing the "Headache Relief Action Plan."

PART 2

NATURAL SOLUTIONS YOUR DOCTOR DOESN'T KNOW

Migraine

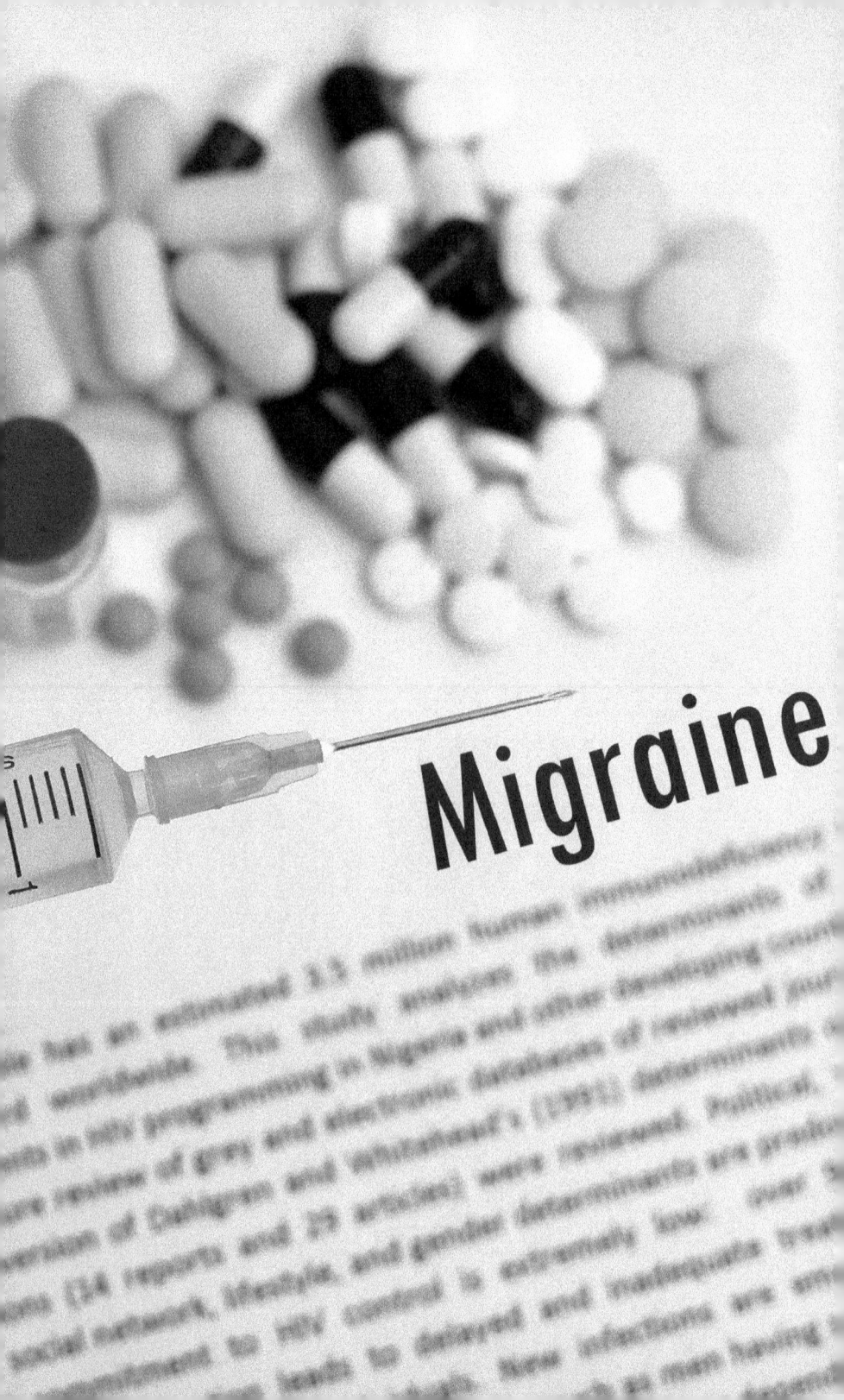

CHAPTER 8

AVOIDING THE PITFALL OF WRONG TREATMENT

Since you are reading this book, I assume you or someone you care for experiences chronic headaches or migraines and are looking for a better quality of life. I also assume that if you're at a point where you're looking for help, you must have gone through your primary care physician, several specialists, and perhaps some alternative medicine options without lasting relief or consistent results. Perhaps you are at a point where you feel nothing can be done or your personal headache situation is hopeless.

Please try not to focus on those negative, helpless feelings if you can; changing the way you think will provide a springboard for more robust results. If you recall from Chapter 4, continuing a treatment plan that is not working is one of the "biggest headache mistakes people make."

There is hope and I am certain more can be done for your condition than you imagine. Why do I think this? Because I have been where you are and I know how doctors and healers think. Therefore, I know the pitfalls of their methods, and I can tell you how to avoid them. Let me explain.

THE COMMON PITFALLS

As odd as it may sound, the reason many healthcare and wellness programs fail is a matter of education. More specifically, I am referring to too much education in one specialty field. You see, when a healthcare practitioner in any field goes from a broad understanding of the human body and illness pathology to a very narrow and specific field, it is like they strap on a set of horse blinders. You know, those dark leather things placed next to the eyes of horses that pull buggies in the street, so they don't get distracted by all the traffic. If you need a heart surgeon, then a specialist is what you want. For general health and wellness, you need a broader view and different perspectives because there usually is not a single root cause to your condition, but many internal and external triggers working together. Let me explain.

If you decide to remain in modern medicine, your options for treating headaches are linked to drugs and injections (more drugs), and, for some, a life of disability. Why? Because modern medicine looks at the body as a biological system needing to be manipulated with drugs to hide its inherent warning signs that something is wrong (i.e., pain, inflammation). I mean, wouldn't you think it silly to just turn up the radio to block out the grinding sound your car engine may be making, rather than fixing the problem causing the sound? The sound is a symptom, an indicator, that something is worn with the vehicle. So masking out the sound with the radio (or taking drugs so you don't feel the headache pain), is not really a sound and lasting solution.

I am not saying that all of the methods used by healthcare providers are not useful or even powerful. I am trying to get you to see how specialists can be blinded by their training in regards to other options and how sticking to one modality at the behest of the others may keep you in pain—especially if that treatment is based on drug therapy. This also holds true for alternative and holistic practices. For the sake of argument and understanding, let's look at a few here.

If you see a chiropractor for pain, they will diagnose and treat you from their perspective. Chiropractors view the spine as the central body part to adjust and keep mobile, supple, and also keep the nerves that protrude from it free and unobstructed. After all, the nerves carry signals to and from the brain, so if they are impinged in some way through subluxation (vertebral misalignment) or muscle spasm (trigger point), they cannot transmit correct information. When this happens, the brain cannot send useful information back to the injured area. The problem here is that not all types of headaches or other chronic pain syndromes are related to the spine or corrected by releasing the impaired spinal nerves.

Acupuncture has a long and illustrious history as China's fabled and powerful healing system. It is based on the theories of meridian (energy) channels and the points of energy that fall along those channels. When the energy is stagnated, deficient or in excess (EDS), its normal flow is hampered and pain or disease develops. By inserting very thin, stainless-steel needles into a selection of points, stagnations can be moved, deficiencies can be strengthened and excesses can be reduced. This leads to free-moving energy in the body, and promotes balance for pain-free existence. However, not all health issues can be traced to an energetic root cause, though parts of them can.

You see, while these wellness methods (and most others) do indeed help people in specific ways, they can only do so within the limits of their specialty, their education, and the healing view of their practitioners. Have you experienced some of these treatments and found good results for a while and then they trailed off? If so, it's because the issues the modality is best suited to treat have been corrected, and the "intractable" or difficult ones are still remaining, unchanged. Many headache and migraine sufferers are left less than enthusiastic with their results.

Everyone, whether doctor or healer, becomes so focused on the theories of their specific healing modality that sometimes they are unable to see the big picture. I saw it because I was looking at the theories of health from the opposite end of the spectrum. I was not only a student, but also a patient who became a healer to find relief from my personal suffering (insider) perspective.

THE HEADACHE RELIEF ACTION PLAN WORKS!

Remember my story about how I became a doctor of Oriental and alternative medicine to cure myself of relentless chronic headaches and found the answer? Here is the amazing part: the answer was simple. So very simple, I began to wonder why no one had discovered it before. And here's my explanation: It was a "can't-see-the-forest-for-the-trees" situation. It required a new way of thinking about the mind, body, and environment. It also required a new way of seeing pain, illness and disease. But once you see it, everything becomes clear.

My search was for a through-line, a single thread connecting all the various theories and modalities that could truly provide me (and later, my patients) with a lasting, proven, life-long way to cure myself. After a decade of trial and error and making left turns on the straight path to wellness, I developed what I passionately refer to as "The Headache Relief Action Plan." It is, at last, a program for real change. I no longer suffer chronic headaches because of it… and neither will you.

THE ESSENCE OF THE PLAN

- ✓ "The Headache Relief Action Plan" works, but you must commit to working it.
- ✓ To live in optimal health, you must learn the essence of how health is derived and maintained.
- ✓ You must strive to have self-compassion.
- ✓ You must become the expert on you and your individual situation.

Before you move on please, once more, ask yourself these personal questions:

- ✓ Do you believe in yourself?
- ✓ Do you believe you can live a happy, healthy, pain-free life?
- ✓ Do you believe that once you understand the method, you can affect your own self-cure?

I believe in it and I believe in you. I know "The Headache Action Plan" works. And I know you can make it work, too. I also know you may think that nothing can be done for you. Yet here you are, reading this book. In your heart and brain, you still hope that something can be done; you have not yet given up all hope. I know you believe you will always have "to manage" your chronic pain, and "live with" your headaches and migraines. Please believe me when I tell you, this simply is not the case.

You see, after I rid myself of my chronic headaches and musculoskeletal pain, I started working out the specifics of how to apply my personal method to hundreds of other health issues. As director of Integrated Energy Medicine, LLC, I gave over 3,000 treatments before moving out of private practice and into patient education, and achieved real and lasting success for my patients.

Right now, you have an idea as to what is wrong with your health because a dozen physicians have labeled it. You just don't know why it is happening to you. You certainly know how much you want to feel great. You just don't know how to get there. "The Headache Relief Action Plan" is your map. You bring questions about your personal health to the table, and this book, as your guide, will tell you the why and show you the how. Together, we will bring the miracle of optimal health into your life.

To be at the point where you are psychologically ready to take control of your health takes great courage and discipline. Are you ready to stop playing the role of victim to ill health and stop being the passive follower of a physician or healer? I am confident you have what it takes to embrace "The Headache Relief Action Plan" and take back control of your life.

Here's to your new life of optimal health and pain-free living. Within that the pages of the next chapters are the answers to the how's, what's and why's to make it happen. We begin with the headache-prevention diet because you can start making real changes by considering the very next thing you choose to put into your mouth. This is followed by natural supplements (herbs, vitamins, minerals, enzymes) that can begin to make changes to your blood, cells, tissues, and inflammation. Next the program offers techniques for stress reduction and for raising oxygen levels in the body through proven meditation and breathing techniques. Proper sleep posture, techniques for overcoming insomnia, and, unique, but powerful, methods for releasing pain-causing, negative thoughts and emotions from your body are taught. From here, you will learn self-stretching techniques for releasing physical tension in the shoulders and neck and learn about different bodywork methods you can use for deeper relief, as along with ancient exercises for restoring balance to the body without causing more headaches. We'll conclude with an overview of energy medicine and how it can help balance and invigorate the body to prevent headaches, and then look at a number of unusual interventions that have been clinically shown to reduce headache and migraine severity. In other words, hang in there because plenty of help, tons of techniques, and advice are up next.

CHAPTER REVIEW

- The wrong approach to headache relief is a dead-end journey that you can avoid.
- Avoiding the pitfalls of incorrect treatment can improve your condition more than you can possibly imagine.
- Many headache programs fail because they are too myopically focused, guided by specialists who are blinded by their education. You now understand how sticking to one treatment modality may be keeping you in pain.
- Specialty methods can help people, but only within limits that aren't right for *everyone*.
- "The Headache Relief Action Plan" helps you understand why you have pain, and what you can do about it.

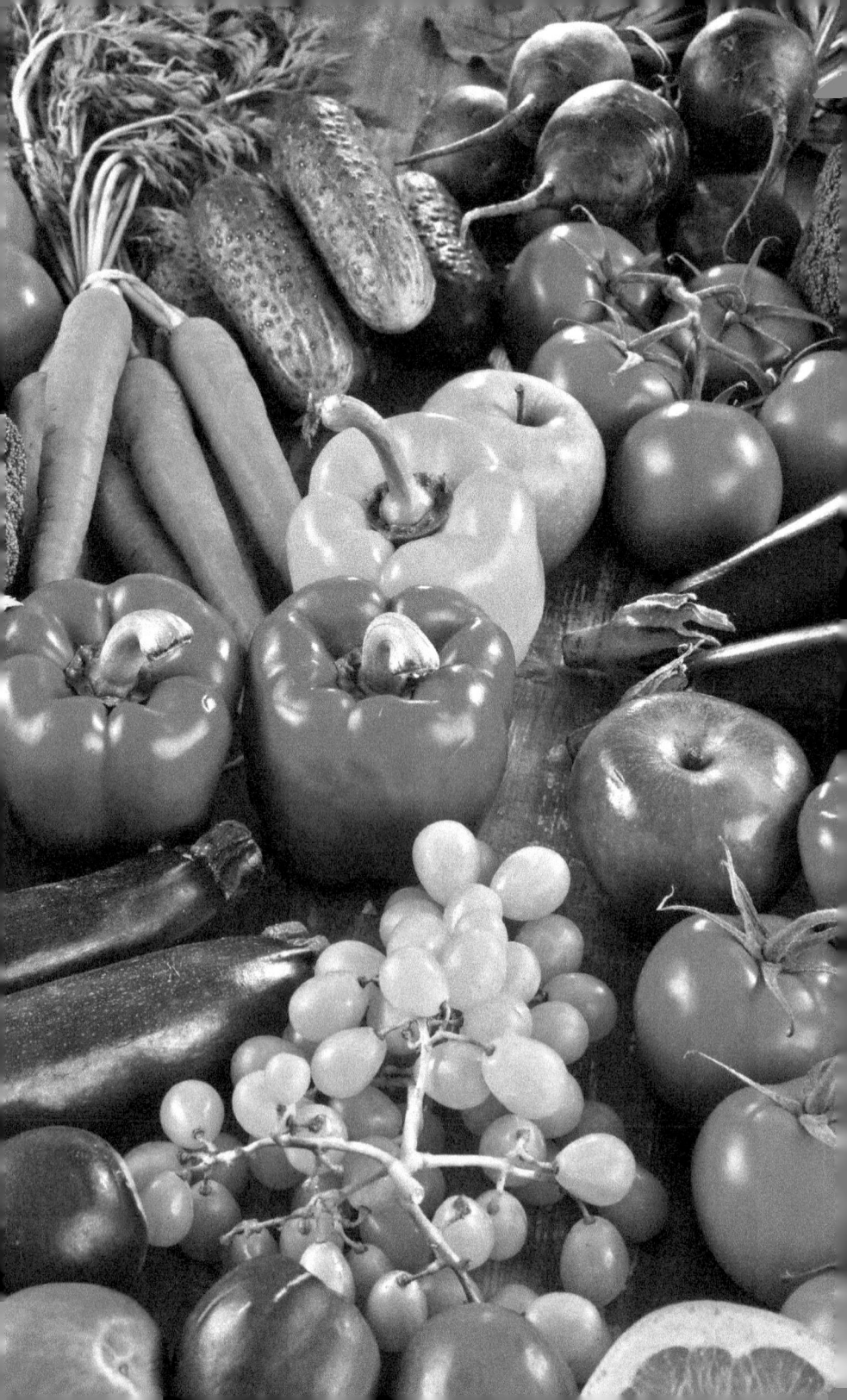

CHAPTER 9

THE HEADACHE PREVENTION DIET

Food is a critical piece of the wellness puzzle, especially when it comes to headaches and migraines. Food can cause pain and inflammation. The typical American diet supports ill health by consisting of an enormous amount of saturated and trans-fats, sugar, processed meats, preservatives, and a frightening amount of processed foods. However, a proper diet that is anti-inflammatory in nature and full of dense nutrients can reduce pain, inflammation and biochemicals to relieve those very symptoms. By switching to an anti-inflammatory diet consisting of healthy whole foods, you can actually decrease inflammation, release biochemicals that affect the vascular and neurological systems, and ease the pain and discomfort associated with headaches and migraines.

The over consumption of a high fat meal accompanied by alcohol and followed by coffee and dessert is a sure way of bringing on a headache in a timely manner. This combination contributes to oxygen deprivation, high blood sugar followed by hypoglycemia, high blood fat, toxins, and caffeine. This kind of diet overtaxes the body in many destructive ways, and the resulting headache is a sign something hazardous has occurred and this kind of feast should be avoided in the future.

For headache sufferers, knowing what, when, and how to eat it is just as important as knowing what to avoid eating. While I do not present specific meal schedules and diet plans here, I do offer general dietary guidelines that will help manage and prevent diet-related headaches from occurring.

THE INFLAMMATION STORY

Pain is generally felt as a reaction to swelling or inflammation in the body. This efferent signal is the body's way of telling you something is wrong and in need of change. Inflammation, then, is both a sign and a symptom of pain.

The term "inflammation" generally evokes thoughts of painful joints and muscles, swelling, and loss of mobility. While these are the obvious markers of inflammation, research also shows that chronic inflammation, if left untreated, can actually lead to serious diseases, including diabetes, heart disease, some cancers, and Alzheimer's!

The amount of inflammation in your body varies and is dependent on a number of factors including your activity level, the amount of sleep you get, the degree of stress in your life, and yes... even the food you eat. What you have to realize is that these factors are cumulative, and build up over time. And the more any or all of these factors get out of control, the more your risk for disease increases.

If you have pain due to inflammation, you may choose to take the traditional medical path, which includes non-steroidal anti-inflammatory drugs (NSAIDs), steroids, and even go so far as having joint-replacement surgery. But none of these "big guns" may be necessary. You should especially avoid long-term use of prescription and over-the-counter anti-inflammatory painkillers. These have been proven to cause liver dysfunction, kidney failure, stomach bleeding and ulcer… all causes of additional inflammation.

Sure, inflammation is a necessary part of the healing process. It brings fluid, nutrients, blood, oxygen, and healing biochemicals to the injured area. However, if left to linger, inflammation poses greater threat to your health, arrests the healing process, and can turn your pain from acute to chronic.

Foods That Cause Pain and Inflammation

When it comes to controlling inflammation, food is a double-edged sword that can both cause and reduce inflammation. There are dozens of foods that create inflammation in our bodies, and there are dozens of foods that reduce and/or prevent inflammation in our bodies. Consuming the right mix of these is essential to living a life of fewer headache onsets and decrease their duration and pain. Here, again, are seven categories of foods that should be avoided if you suffer chronic headaches and migraines.

1. **Animal Milk Products** (Milk, Cream, Ice Cream, Cheese, Cottage Cheese, Yogurt)
2. **Hydrogenated oils** (Non-Dairy Creamer, Crackers, Cookies, Chips, Snack Bars)
3. **Nitrates** (Hot Dogs, Cold Cuts, Pepperoni, Sausage, Bacon, Liverwurst)
4. **Processed Sugars** (Candy, Soda, Bread, Bottled Fruit Juice, Cookies, Snack Bars)

5. **Nightshades** (Potatoes, Peppers, Tomatoes, Eggplant, Paprika)
6. **Convenience Foods** (French Fries, Onion Rings, Loaded Baked Potatoes, Fatty Burgers, Mexican Food, Pizza, Calzones, Stromboli)
7. **Processed White Foods** (Flour, Bread, Pasta, Pizza, Crackers, Pretzels, Donuts)

Are you surprised?

As you can see, most of the items on this list are actually the staple American diet. Is it any wonder Americans are among the most obese and pain suffering people in the world? If you look closely at this list, you will notice these ingredients are found in just about every snack, frozen dinner, bread and even so-called "healthy" foods. Whatever you do, don't believe the marketing. Read the labels instead.

Do yourself an easy, no-cost favor… stop eating foods from the above list if you have inflamed joints or are in pain. Merely eliminating these items from your diet will help stop the inflammation cycle when its natural course has run. By eating these foods, you are increasing the longevity of the inflammation, and thus self-inducing your own chronic pain. Now that you know which foods actually cause inflammation or make it worse, let's look at the foods that can help reduce and even prevent inflammation.

Foods That REDUCE Pain and Inflammation

We all know the food we eat is our primary source of nutrients and energy, and becomes the substance of our blood. In addition to oxygen and water, food is the substance of life. Food can make you strong and keep you in homeostatic balance. A diet high in fiber and whole foods, low in preservatives and unhealthy fat, and infused with blood-invigorating aromatic spices can help reduce pain and inflammation.

It is essential to any healthful diet – especially a diet to prevent headaches and migraines – that you consume as much fresh, organic, whole foods as possible. Eating foods in or as close to their original state is one of the keys to being healthy. It also prevents self-induced, diet-based inflammation and pain. Here is a list of the best foods known to prevent and help reduce inflammation and pain. These should be eaten throughout the day as part of balanced, wholesome meals:

- Wild Alaskan salmon
- Fresh whole fruits
- Bright colored vegetables (*except nightshades)
- Green and white tea
- Purified and distilled water
- Healthy oils (olive, flax, hemp, safflower, hazelnut, coconut)
- Beef and poultry that is certified organic
- Nuts, legumes, and seeds
- Dark green leafy vegetables
- Organic oatmeal (regular, not instant)
- Aromatic spices (turmeric, ginger, cloves, garlic, onion, coriander, ground mustard seed)

As you can see, a diet high in whole foods and low in preservatives and unhealthy fat is the key to an essential part of a headache and migraine relief plan. Not only do the above-listed foods actually work to reduce pain and inflammation, but they also support proper nerve function, muscle, and bone health.

Remember, the acid/alkaline or pH level of your body (which can cause or prevent inflammation) is related to the food you consume. Using the following chart, see how what you consume on a daily or monthly basis may be contributing to the worsening of your headaches and migraines.

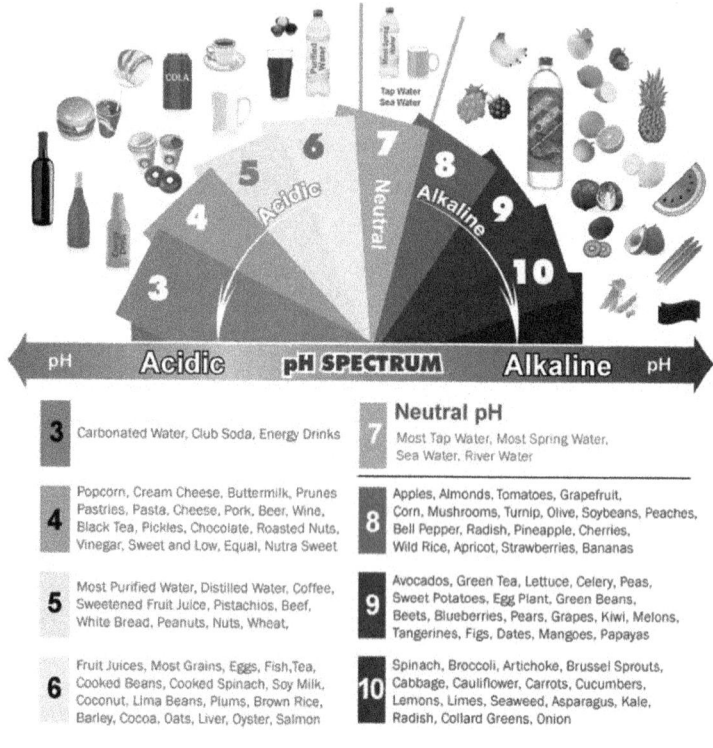

pH	Acidic		pH	Neutral / Alkaline
3	Carbonated Water, Club Soda, Energy Drinks		7	Neutral pH — Most Tap Water, Most Spring Water, Sea Water, River Water
4	Popcorn, Cream Cheese, Buttermilk, Prunes, Pastries, Pasta, Cheese, Pork, Beer, Wine, Black Tea, Pickles, Chocolate, Roasted Nuts, Vinegar, Sweet and Low, Equal, Nutra Sweet		8	Apples, Almonds, Tomatoes, Grapefruit, Corn, Mushrooms, Turnip, Olive, Soybeans, Peaches, Bell Pepper, Radish, Pineapple, Cherries, Wild Rice, Apricot, Strawberries, Bananas
5	Most Purified Water, Distilled Water, Coffee, Sweetened Fruit Juice, Pistachios, Beef, White Bread, Peanuts, Nuts, Wheat,		9	Avocados, Green Tea, Lettuce, Celery, Peas, Sweet Potatoes, Egg Plant, Green Beans, Beets, Blueberries, Pears, Grapes, Kiwi, Melons, Tangerines, Figs, Dates, Mangoes, Papayas
6	Fruit Juices, Most Grains, Eggs, Fish, Tea, Cooked Beans, Cooked Spinach, Soy Milk, Coconut, Lima Beans, Plums, Brown Rice, Barley, Cocoa, Oats, Liver, Oyster, Salmon		10	Spinach, Broccoli, Artichoke, Brussel Sprouts, Cabbage, Cauliflower, Carrots, Cucumbers, Lemons, Limes, Seaweed, Asparagus, Kale, Radish, Collard Greens, Onion

credit: mindbodygreen.com[1]

Let's now look into the direct role that fiber, water, and the glycemic index of food play in triggering, reducing and preventing headaches and migraines.

FIBER AND HEADACHE

To begin, dietary fiber is so important in headache prevention that it should be an essential part of your diet. Fiber keeps the bowels functioning properly for efficient elimination, stabilizes blood sugar levels, and clears fats from the blood stream. The American Dietetic Association and the American Cancer Society have both recommended we consume from 25-to-30 grams of fiber daily, which is abundant in plant products such as fruits, grains, and vegetables.

There are two forms of fiber: soluble and insoluble. Soluble fiber such as pectin (found in most fruits) dissolves easily in water so it can be absorbed in the intestine and circulate in the blood stream. Soluble fiber in the blood has the ability to attach itself to blood fats and create a complex that will remove these fats from the blood system, and lower cholesterol.

Insoluble fiber absorbs in water also, but it is not absorbed in the intestine. It remains there and forms the majority of bulk necessary to "sweep" bodily wastes through the intestine and out of the body. Without fiber, the colon cannot effectively move toxic waste products from the body, allowing stools to putrefy, and toxins to circulate back into the blood stream.

In addition to fiber, seeds and grains are the gold mines of minerals, especially calcium, phosphorus, magnesium, and iron. They contain most of the vitamins, particularly vitamins A, B and E. They are nature's best source of unsaturated fatty acids and lecithin. They are excellent sources of protein.

WATER AND HEADACHE

It is vital that every human being drink copious amounts of water every day—especially those who suffer headaches. Since water makes up roughly 75% or three-fourths of the human body (and 85% of the brain), it only makes sense that no tissue, organ or gland can function properly without ample supply of this natural fluid. It is the improper functioning of the digestive system, lungs, liver, and kidneys that not only contributes to and triggers headaches, but make us ill. Indeed, humans cannot exist without the magic elixir known as water, which, next to oxygen, is the most vital substance on Earth.

Drinking ample quantities of water every day is so important that for centuries many traditional cultures have engaged its healing qualities to cure and prevent various illnesses and diseases. Traditional Chinese medicine, for example, recognized the healing powers of water more than 3,000 years ago. Even Hippocrates, the father of modern medicine, was said to have drank and bathed in water to benefit from the healing properties of its mineral content. Indeed, the mere consumption of this fluid can help restore the body to its natural state of homeostasis by clearing toxins, cleansing the colon, flushing the liver and kidneys, and emptying the bowels—all necessary elements to removing and preventing a number of headaches.

Why Dehydration Causes Headaches

With the abundance of water available in the United States and the sheer necessity of it to our health and well-being, it is a wonder that the many illnesses and ailments—including headaches—are actually caused or aggravated by simple dehydration. The leading researcher of our time on illness and disease caused by dehydration is Dr. F. Batmanghelidj, an internist trained at St. Mary's Hospital Medical School of London University, and, one of the last students of Sir Alexander Flemming, the discoverer of penicillin. In his book, *The Body's Many Cries for Water*, Dr. Batmanghelidj asserts that "Chronic, unintentional dehydration is the origin of most pain and degenerative diseases in the human body."[2] These, he notes, include migraines.

Batmanghelidj found that as the water content of tissues falls to a certain point due to dehydration, the bi-layer membranes that surround cells contract, forming a barrier that prevents further water loss. This obstructs the free movement of molecules, so that metabolism and elimination are limited. Slow metabolism and elimination lead to the build-up of toxins in the blood, which can manifest as a chemical-induced headache.

It is important to understand that regardless of the quantity of your daily water intake, its percentage in urine remains constant at around 95%. When the hypothalamus detects a lowering of water volume in the body, it signals the pituitary gland to release the anti-diuretic hormone (ADH) into the bloodstream, which increases the capacity of the kidneys to reabsorb and recycle water. In essence, when the body moves into survival mode by contracting the bi-layer membranes, the kidneys keep recycling and concentrating the urine in an effort to maintain sufficient hydration. Thus, the less water put into the body, the less the body's ability to cleanse itself of poisonous toxins through elimination via urine, feces, perspiration, and the breath. And since waste products that are left to accumulate in your tissues create chronic pain, headaches, and many diseases, water intake is necessary to facilitate the effective elimination of toxic build-up.

The effects of overeating foods containing nitrates, toxic chemicals, excess sugars and/or alcohol overtaxes the colon and causes one to experience exhaustion, lethargy, unending, dull headaches, and makes them susceptible to catching colds easily or becomes seriously ill. It is precisely the absorption of the nutrients in the colon and intestines from the food we eat that prevent, cause or cure what ails us. In fact, research has indicated that a thorough flushing of the mucus folds in the colonic tract where toxins and wastes generally remain will cleans the system and keep the body healthy and the immune system strong. At the same time, quantities of water are known to revitalize the kidney and liver. Thus, by drinking ample quantities of water, the colon will become more effective, thus increasing the quantity and supply of fresh blood that can then move throughout the body. Improper blood flow and insulin levels are known migraine triggers.

In short, it is vital that your cells, tissues, and organs be sufficiently hydrated for your body to maintain its natural state of homeostasis. It is only in this state that the chemical toxins, which have built up in the body can be properly processed and eliminated. Water is the only substance that can properly hydrate the body; not caffeinated coffees and teas, carbonated sodas or sugar-filled fruit drinks. Only water, pure and simple as it is, will keep you healthy and help the body eliminate many of the underlying headache triggers.

How Much Water Is Enough?

There is much written about the specific quantities of water required for the body to function properly. Certainly, drinking a single glass of water at lunch or dinner will not do the job. And while the FDA recommends six, 8-ounce glasses of water per day, other experts suggest we need to consume 8 ounces per day for every 20 pounds of body weight.

However, trying to remember specific times and quantities of water to consume can be cumbersome. I personally ascribe to a more liberal method of drinking water all day and watching my urine color as a gauge for when I need to consume more water. It is generally agreed that adults need at least two quarts of water per day under ideal conditions—and colas, coffee, and iced tea do not count toward this. If you drink water from a bottle throughout the day, after a period of hydration, you will find yourself making frequent trips to the restroom to relieve yourself. A continuous flow of water through your body to continually wash away toxins in your system and prevent them from building up and triggering headaches is exactly what you want.

If you maintain a constant flow of water through your body, your kidneys will not become over-taxed and forced to concentrate urine in an effort to maintain proper levels of hydration in your body. When urine is concentrated as a result of dehydration, its color becomes dark. Therefore, if you find yourself drinking throughout the day, but it has been a while since your last glass, check your urine. If it is colored, it is a sign that you are becoming dehydrated—and this happens quickly when consuming caffeinated diuretic beverages like coffee and soda—and it is time for another glass or two of water. I always keep my bottle of spring or filtered water filled and at my side. This way, I never forget to drink from it, and I'm not forced to consume chemically treated tap water.

The undeniable fact is that next to air, water is the most vital substance known to man. Keeping the body properly hydrated helps remove toxins from the body while maintaining proper blood flow and organ, muscle and glandular functions. It is best to drink water at room temperature so as not to shock the system. Remember, drinking water throughout the day, as dictated by urine color, is the best way to maintain proper hydration.

Your body will never feel as light or as clean and unpolluted as it does when it is properly hydrated. And in the process, a large portion of the on-going headache triggers that attacked you in the past will be eliminated.

Not All Water is Safe to Drink

Not all water is suitable for drinking. In fact, in cities such as Baltimore, the fecal level in the water supply has been so high that the government had to step in and deem the situation a state of emergency. Then, there is the horrendous water supply in Flint, Michigan with natural gas blending with their water from old pipelines and fracking.

As Drs. Milne and More note in their *Definitive Guide to Headaches*:

> "...even with a filter, tap water is not the safest to drink, especially if you are headache-prone...With every cup of tap water you swallow, you increase your risk of being exposed to heavy metals and/or chemical toxins, especially if you fill your glass during the times the water districts add any of the 700 chemicals available for use in water supply."[3]

According to a report published by the Environmental Protection Agency (EPA):

> "Naturally occurring contaminants also are being found in drinking water. For example, the radioactive gas radon-222 is found in certain types of rock and can get into ground water. People can be exposed to radon in water by drinking it, while showering, or when washing dishes."[4]

With this in mind, it is best that headache sufferers not drink water directly from their tap, as natural and chemical toxin build-up in the blood stream is a definite—though preventable—headache trigger. Thus, drinking purified bottled or filtered water should be the only option.

Avoid Toxic Water Bottles and Packaging

Researchers Nancy Berman and Lydia Vermeer at Kansas University (KU) Medical Center[5] had a hypothesis they wanted to test. Since more women than men get migraines, and they often are related to the menstrual cycle, perhaps hormones play a key role in migraines. They also wondered if bisphenol A (BPA), a hormone-disrupting chemical used to make plastic firm, might play a part. BPA leaks into food and drinks from food and beverage containers. When you consume BPA, the chemical acts like estrogen.

Does BPA, then, also trigger migraines?

To put this hypothesis to the test, they injected lab rats with BPA and found that the BPA activated estrogen receptors. The lab animals also displayed significantly worse headache symptoms than animals not exposed to BPA.

"We're hypothesizing that people with migraines do not have more BPA in their system, but that they're more sensitive to BPA," Vermeer said. "Many people with migraines are more sensitive to changes in things like estrogen."

While the Food and Drug Administration has declared BPA to be safe in low levels, it has also expressed concern about deleterious effects on the brain and behavior and in the prostate health of young children and even fetuses. As such, the FDA has banned the use of BPA from baby bottles and plastic nipples.

Hmmm, sounds "unsafe" to me! To boot, Canada, France, and China have actually banned BPA from many consumer applications.

BPA is found in water bottles, including those with recycle codes 3 and 7, and also in the lining of many canned goods. The dilemma with this is that one of the preventive measures of migraines is to drink plenty of water and most plastic water bottles contain the harmful BPA chemical. So, that's a real problem.

The new solution: Drink filtered water out of an aluminum-free, metal container or a glass or plastic bottle, which is marked "BPA Free." I do. And while we don't yet have clear proof of human reaction to BPA, as we do with rats, it takes no money and little effort to prevent a migraine by changing the type of vessel from which we consume our water. So, the good news here is that we are now aware of another potential migraine trigger (BPA), and we can easily avoid it by purchasing canned goods and food and beverages in plastic containers that are marked BPA-free or have recycling code #2.

BLOOD SUGAR AND GLYCEMIC LOAD

More important than individual calorie and fat content of food is its glycemic load, or how quickly or slowly the body breaks down food, converts it into sugar and either uses it for fuel or stores it as fat.

A chart of glycemic loads is listed below for each food based on its relative glycemic ratio of fiber to sugar content. The more a food is processed or has had sugar added, the higher its numerical index. In contrast, the higher its whole grain content, the lower its index number.

GLYCEMIC INDEX CHART
Low Glycemic (55 or Below)   High Glycemic (70 or Higher)

SNACKS	G.I.	STARCH	G.I.	VEGETABLES	G.I.	FRUITS	G.I.	DAIRY	G.I.
Pizza	33	Bagel, Plain	33	Broccoli	10	Cherries	22	Yogurt, Plain	14
Chocolate Bar	49	White Rice	38	Pepper	10	Apple	38	Yogurt, Low Fat	14
Pound Cake	54	White Spaghetti	38	Lettuce	10	Orange	43	Whole Milk	30
Popcorn	55	Sweet Potato	44	Mushrooms	10	Grapes	46	Soy Milk	31
Energy Bar	58	White Bread	49	Onions	10	Kiwi	52	Skim Milk	32
Soda	72	Brown Rice	55	Green Peas	48	Banana	56	Chocolate Milk	35
Doughnut	76	Pancakes	67	Carrots	49	Pineapple	66	Yogurt, Fruit	36
Jelly Beans	80	Wheat Bread	80	Beets	64	Watermelon	72	Custard	43
Pretzels	83	Baked Potato	85	Onions	75	Dates	103	Ice Cream	60

Many individuals who struggle with weight do so because of problems with blood sugar, insulin resistance, and metabolic issues that can be controlled by maintaining a glycemic load of 50 points or lower per day. In this way, you fill your meals with food that breaks down slowly into sugars in your body and, therefore, do not promote too much insulin release and storage of sugars as fats.

Ideally, you want to break down your food slowly and use it as fuel as you go. Weight gain happens when the body stores unused food as fat or when too much insulin is released as a reaction to eating too many simple carbohydrates.

Look at the glycemic load chart above and consider how your daily eating habits are directly responsible for your weight issues, in addition to associated health issues like type 2 diabetes, metabolic syndrome, and insulin resistance syndrome. If you eat whole foods and look to food as fuel for life-force, and not for weight loss, you can level off at a healthy weight by eating healthfully and not triggering an over-release of insulin from poor food choices.

WHEN AND HOW TO EAT

Now that we know what *not* to consume and what to include in our diets, let's look at how and when to eat. On a fundamental level, we need to eat to live, and the activation of hypoglycemia is a known cause of headaches. Along with under-eating, overeating also causes headaches. It is therefore essential that the headache sufferer eat frequent, smaller meals to prevent headaches due to over-consumption of food and imbalances in blood sugar levels. I recommend eating one-third sized portions every three hours in an effort to keep energy levels high and blood sugar and serotonin levels stabilized.

As you can see, there are numerous headache triggers associated with diet, body chemicals, and headaches. And every one of them is related to lifestyle choices. Follow a healthy eating program high in fruits, vegetables, and complex carbohydrates.

Avoid caffeine, refined sugar, simple carbohydrates, tyramine-containing foods, and alcohol. Eat frequently, chew your food well, and don't drink too much during meal time. Following this straightforward approach to eating, will remove the headache triggers directly linked with diet from your life.

CHAPTER REVIEW

- Food is a critical piece of the wellness puzzle, especially when it comes to chronic headaches.
- Specific foods and food groups can cause pain, inflammation, and chemical imbalances in the body, which trigger headaches.
- The typical American diet – filled with saturated and trans-fats, sugars, preservatives, convenience food, and overly processed foods – is a deadly recipe for acidity, inflammation, and pain.
- Avoid inflammatory foods and consume as much fresh, organic, whole foods as possible.
- Eating a diet rich in anti-inflammatory foods, filled with dense nutrients, can reduce pain, inflammation, and body mass.
- Essential, yet often overlooked foods like green tea, mushrooms, turmeric, and water are proven to reduce inflammation and pain.
- When eating for headache prevention, forget diets, counting carbs, and calories. Stick to the basics of healthy eating. Stabilize your blood sugar by knowing the glycemic load of everything you eat, and consume more alkaline and metabolism boosting foods and spices.

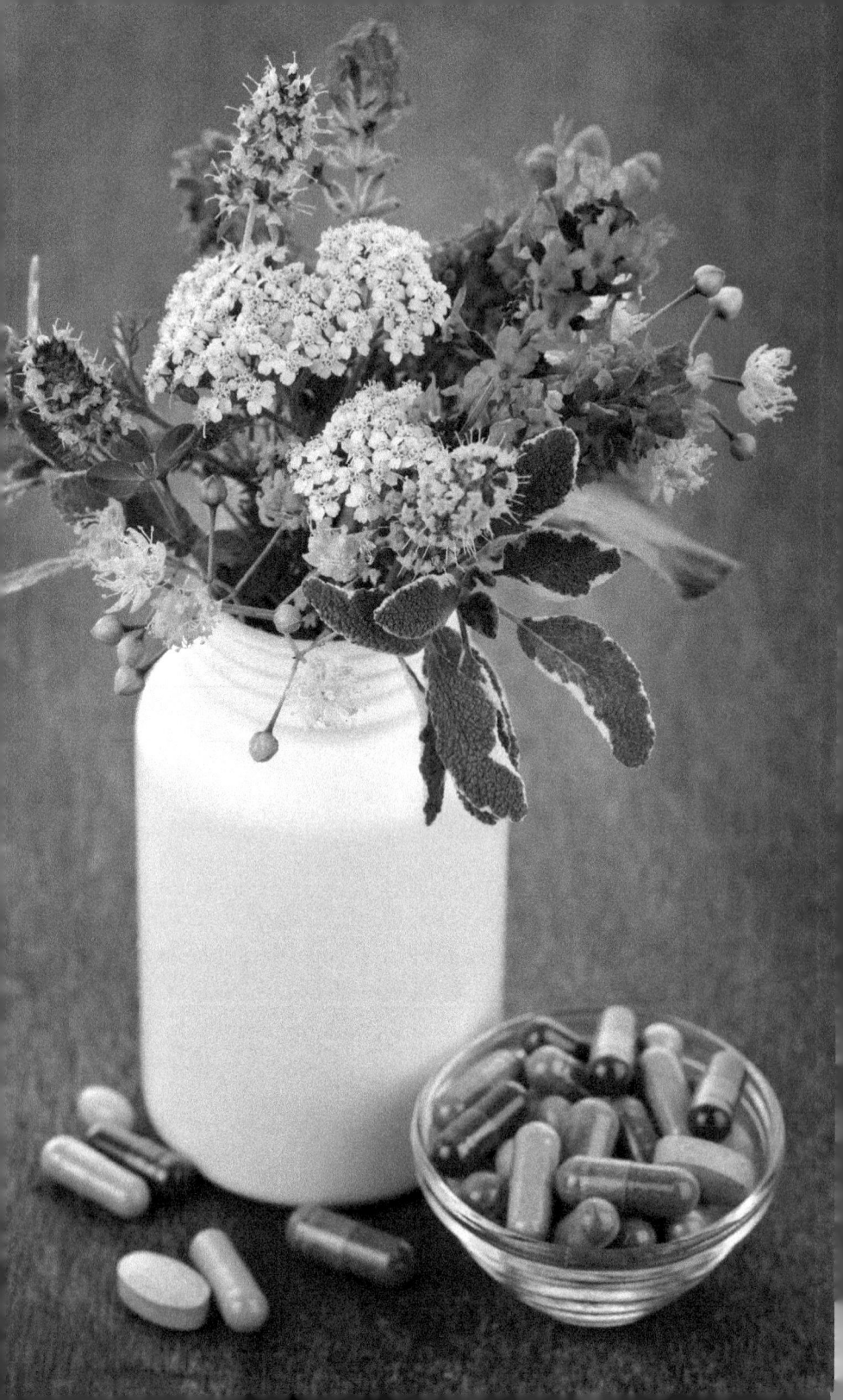

CHAPTER 10

SUPPLEMENTS FOR HEADACHE RELIEF AND PREVENTION

Americans spend millions of dollars annually on analgesics, anti-inflammatories, beta blockers, calcium channel blockers, triptans, and other medical chemicals to help stave off and reduce the pain and symptoms associated with headaches.

While drugs, both prescribed and over-the-counter, are the most popular remedy for headaches and migraines, they may not be the most effective; and they certainly are not without side effects. Natural vitamins and nutritional supplements, in some cases, have been shown to be just as effective (and some more effective) than their lab-produced counterparts.

Herbs, Vitamins, and Minerals

This chapter begins by stressing the fact that natural supplements are not the same as chemically manufactured medicines. To begin with, they are made of natural ingredients and are less toxic, and, therefore, less harmful to the body in the recommended doses if taken as directed. Even in low doses, many prescription and over-the-counter drugs are toxic and have short-term negative effects on the liver, kidney, and gastro-intestinal (GI) tract. When taken over the long term or not as directed, pharma meds can cause serious organ damage. Why?

Because drugs are created in a lab and our bodies are not equipped to digest and process them. Moreover, drugs are super powerful, which gives them the ability to offer fast relief of symptoms, like pain and inflammation. This is good for short-term use, but can be harmful over time. The body just can't metabolize these drugs sufficiently to prevent them from causing new damage and side effects.

Natural supplements, on the other hand, are made from the stuff of nature. This includes leaves, twigs, berries, bark, roots, vines, vitamins, and minerals. They are natural substances that can't be regulated by the FDA because they are technically foodstuffs. If you understood herbology, you could, as many traditional cultures do, adjust your diet to include beneficial herbs in your meals. However, for painful conditions, such as acute and chronic headaches and migraines, this would mean taking them at every meal. Taking these ingredients as supplements to your diet is the way to go.

In addition to the other methods and strategies discussed in this book, I recommend taking natural supplements to reduce pain and inflammation and reduce the onset of neuro-vascular changes without side effects. In the following paragraphs, I offer an overview of dozens of different natural supplements shown to help reduce and prevent headaches. Read each, keeping in mind your specific condition and how some may be more effective for you than others.

BOSWELLIA SERRATA

Boswellia serrata is a traditional Indian Ayurvedic remedy for inflammatory conditions. It is extracted from the gum of the Indian boswellia tree and has been in use for centuries to treat joint pain and inflammation. It provides anti-inflammatory activity in areas where there is chronic inflammation by turning off the pro-inflammatory cytokines that begin the inflammatory process. Moreover, research shows that the acids contained within boswellia extract stop the formation of immune cells known as leukotrienes, which are responsible for inflammation. This property allows blood to flow unobstructed to the joints for healing and improved mobility.

BURDOCK ROOT

Burdock root is a natural botanical that is used widely for many conditions, among them arthritic pain, swollen joints, and rheumatism. More than anything else, clinical studies have found it most effective as a blood purifier that helps rid the body of deleterious toxins and clear congestion from the circulatory, lymphatic, respiratory, and urinary systems. Burdock is said to cleanse and eliminate long-term impurities from the blood very rapidly through its action on both the liver and kidneys. For those who suffer from chronic headaches and have taken too much Tylenol, burdock root has been clinical proven to protect liver cells from the damage of taking acetaminophen. It is believed to stimulate the gallbladder and encourage liver cells to regenerate.

BUTTERBUR

Butterbur (Petasites hybridus) is a perennial shrub that is effective for people suffering from migraines (without aura) when taken for four months at 75 mg, two times a day. It acts like a beta-blocker in the body, reducing inflammation, controlling blood pressure, and balancing blood flow to the brain.

The latest American Academy of Neurology/American Headache Society guidelines published an "outline of effective treatments" in the *Journal of Neuropsychiatric Disease and Treatment*.[1] The guidelines listed effective treatments for preventing migraine attacks and lessening their severity, and butterbur was included. A 2004 study showed the best response after three months with a 58% reduction in attacks. A significant 71% of the nearly 250 people in the study responded positively to the supplement.

Because some butterbur treatments contain chemicals (pyrrolizidine alkaloids), which can cause damage to the liver, it is important to choose only products that are certified and carry a "PA-free" label.

FEVERFEW

Feverfew (Tanacetum parthenium) has been studied more than any other supplement for its effects on migraine. It has been shown to help reduce the frequency and severity of migraines in those who take 100 mg daily. Feverfew works by relaxing blood vessels and decreasing inflammation, thereby improving blood circulation in the brain.

OMEGA-3 FATTY ACIDS

The omega-3 fatty acids found in abundance in fish oil derived from cod, trout, herring, salmon, and other cold-water fish are proven to reduce inflammation. Research from Cardiff University in Great Britain found that cod liver oil not only relieves pain, but also stops and even reverses the damage caused by osteoarthritis and rheumatoid arthritis. Omega-3s help morning stiffness, regenerate joint tissue, and have been shown to also aid in autoimmune disease like Rheumatoid Arthritis (RA), lupus, and psoriasis.

Omega-3 fatty acids are one of the most powerful and natural anti-inflammatories that have been shown to reduce the frequency, duration, and severity of migraines. The three fatty acids in fish oil are known as ALA, DHA, and EPA. Taking a combined dose of 1,000 mg daily can help with a host of issues, including headaches and migraines.

RUTIN

Rutin is a flavonoid composed of the flavonol quercetin and the disaccharide rutinose. Rutin is found naturally in a variety of plants, and dietary sources including black tea and apple peels. Rutin's anti-inflammatory potential is attributed mainly to its powerful antioxidant activity. Rutin also helps maintain the levels of reduced glutathione, which is a powerful biological antioxidant. The combination of these activities helps to minimize the cellular damage and resulting inflammation caused by the various oxidative processes.

SAMe (S-ADENOSYL METHIONINE)

SAMe is one of the natural chemicals made within the body that science has been able to duplicate in a lab, and make into a supplement. Studies have shown SAMe supplementation to be comparable to the pain-relieving effects of Celebrex by the second month of taking the product, but without the side effects. The SAMe chemical has a role in pain, depression, liver disease, and has been shown effective when used for relieving the symptoms of migraine headaches, osteoarthritis, fibromyalgia, bursitis, Alzheimer's disease, multiple sclerosis (MS), depression and more.

TURMERIC (CURCUMIN)

In traditional cultures that are thousands of years old, like India, there are deep traditions of cooking daily meals with medicinal roots and herbs. Turmeric is one such medicinal root that has made its way into a vast number of Indian recipes.

Studies have shown that the antioxidant properties of curcumin, the active component of turmeric, are able to reduce COX-2 – an inflammatory enzyme. Usually anti-inflammatory medications like aspirin and NSAIDs are prescribed for a migraine. Laboratory studies and clinical research have found that turmeric and the phenolics compounds in it have anti-inflammatory and antioxidant properties. This is similar to steroid medications like indomethacin. Hence, it has been suggested that turmeric could be used as a supportive treatment for migraines.

Dr. Leigh Erin Connealy of Newport Natural Health recommends using turmeric to treat cluster headaches. Cluster headaches are those that occur on a chronic basis and might recur frequently for more than a week. Typical causes of cluster headaches include your diet and environmental issues. Take a dose of up to 500 milligrams of turmeric as many as three times a day as a preventive measure, not only when you have pain. Many health food stores sell turmeric pills or you can buy the spice in bulk and make your own pills by filling gel capsules.

Unlike aspirin or ibuprofen, turmeric's curcumin reduces inflammation naturally without damaging the liver or kidneys. It has been found especially helpful in treating conditions like arthritis, sports injuries, irritable bowel syndrome, Crohn's disease, tendinitis, and various autoimmune diseases. Some research even suggests that curcumin may also help those suffering asthma, inflammatory bowel disease, and, yes, even cancer.

The thing is, you just can't get enough turmeric in your diet to stave off headaches. So it is recommended that you purchase turmeric or curcumin supplements, and take 500 mg up to three times a day as a preventive measure or on days when you feel a headache may strike.

WHITE WILLOW BARK

Since the time of Hippocrates, white willow bark has been in use as a natural means of reducing inflammation and pain, specifically associated with headaches, osteoarthritis, rheumatoid arthritis, as well as, backaches, gout and PMS. The bark of the willow tree contains the chemical salicin, which has a similar effect in the body as acetylsalicylic acid (aspirin). But it's better than aspirin because it has none of the gastrointestinal side effects, and it naturally contains flavonoids (anti-inflammatory compounds found in plants).

KUDZU

Kudzu is a Japanese and Chinese vine whose roots are rich in isoflavones, such as puerarin, daidzein, and daidzin. A report published in the journal *Headache* found kudzu effective for treating cluster headaches.[2] According to the report, 69% of headache respondents who took kudzu experienced decreased intensity of attacks; 56% of respondents had decreased frequency: and, 31% had decreased duration with minimal side effects.

LAVENDER

Lavender has been a go-to remedy for everything from insomnia and anxiety to post-surgical pain and headaches. Lavender consists of linalool and linalyl acetate, which effectively reduce excitation of the nervous system. As such, lavender effectively induces relaxation, reduces inflammation and the stress response, and acts as a sedative, thereby acting as an analgesic to reduce pain. This makes lavender great for treating stress, anxiety and headaches.

LEMONGRASS

Australian lemongrass has been used by traditional healers "down under" for possibly thousands of years. And in the recent study published in the journal, *Evidence-based Complementary and Alternative Medicine*, lemongrass was found in tests to inhibit the clumping of human blood platelets in a similar fashion to the way aspirin does. Scientists from Griffith University recently released the results of a five-year study on the plant, which showed it is capable of relieving headaches and migraines. They found that Australian lemongrass could be as "good as aspirin when it comes to treating headaches." Lemongrass is tasty in food, and found in Southeast Asian cuisines, and can also be drank as a tea.

MELATONIN

Melatonin as a supplement is a lab-created form of the natural hormone produced by the pineal gland. It has been shown as an effective aid for insomnia. However, the National Sleep Foundation reports that "when scientists conduct tests to compare melatonin as a "sleeping pill" to a placebo, most studies show no benefit of melatonin." Evidence that melatonin can reset the body clock is more well established, although it is not clear whether exposure to light may be more effective."[3]

The results of a randomized, double-blind, placebo-controlled study published in the May 2016 issue of *the Journal of Neurology, Neurosurgery & Psychology*[4] compared the effects of taking 3 mg of melatonin at bedtime versus 25 mg of Amitriptyline once daily over a 12-week period for migraine prevention.

Amitriptyline is a tricyclic antidepressant, perhaps better known by its brand names Elavil, Vanatrip, and Endep. It is most commonly used to treat depression by affecting a balance of chemicals in the brain that, when imbalanced, cause symptoms of depression. It has also come into its own as a drug to treat migraines. The bad news for Amitriptyline is its major side effects, which include: chest pain or discomfort, convulsions, difficulty in breathing, inability to move arms, legs, or facial muscles, inability to speak, loss of consciousness, mental depression or anxiety, seizures, and severe muscle stiffness, among others!

At the end of the three-month study, those taking melatonin experienced a reduction of 2.7 "headache days," where the Amitriptyline groups saw a smaller reduction of 2.2 headache days during the same period. The placebo group found a reduction of 1.1 headache days. What's more, the study also found:

- ✓ Melatonin was superior to amitriptyline in the percentage of patients with a greater than 50% reduction in migraine frequency.
- ✓ Melatonin was better tolerated than amitriptyline.
- ✓ Weight loss was found in the melatonin group; a slight weight gain in placebo and significantly for amitriptyline users.

For those who do not get headaches frequently and may only get a migraine twice per month with each lasting for 2-6 days, the reduction in "headache days" is as significant as the reduction of headache onset. If you suffer migraines and maybe insomnia, go ahead and take melatonin before bed every night and see how it works for you.

VITAMINS

Vitamins are essential to health. Every natural thing you eat contains the vitamins your body needs for growth, repair, bone density, pH balance, and hormone regulation. The problem is that many people don't have access to organic whole foods, so vitamin supplementation is important. When suffering from headaches and migraines, the following vitamins may help:

Vitamin A helps decrease levels of blood fat, while helping to maintain health of the skin and glands.

Folic Acid/Folate (a B vitamin) helps metabolize homocysteine (a migraine trigger), supports the production of red blood cells and proper nerve function. Helps stave off some cancers, stroke, heart attack, anemia, and migraine. In addition to supplements and fortified breads and cereals, good sources of folic acid include beans (lima, pinto, navy, garbanzo), lentils, spinach, collard greens, and turnip greens.

Vitamin B2 (riboflavin) is essential for proper functioning of vitamins B6 and B3, and helps metabolize carbohydrates, fats and proteins, while also helping to convert tryptophan to niacin. Vitamin B2 supports the production of cellular energy. B2 is an antioxidant that helps protect cells from free-radical oxygen damage and is a key component in the process of converting food to energy. As a supplement taken for three months at 400 mg per day, studies showed it reduced migraine onset by 50 percent in more than half the people who take it. In addition to fortified grains, breads and cereals, riboflavin is found in lean meats, eggs, grass-fed cow's milk, yogurt, collard greens and other green leafy vegetables, nuts, legumes, and cremini mushrooms.

Vitamin B3 (niacin) helps lower blood fat.

Vitamin B6 (pyridoxine) helps produce serotonin from tryptophan, and helps metabolize fats. It produces antibodies and expedites the conversion of glycogen to glucose. Vitamin B6 works to stave off migraines by supporting a broad number of activities in your nervous system by breaking down sugars and starches, and metabolizing homocysteine. In addition to taking a supplement, food sources include avocados, bananas, beans, sunflower seeds, spinach, potatoes, tuna, cod, halibut, liver, chicken, turkey, and eggs.

Vitamin B12 is a nutrient that promotes healthy blood cells, prevents anemia, and fights off inflammation of the joints and helps make DNA. It is essential for the normal functioning of the cells, nervous system, and gastrointestinal tract.

Vitamin B12 supports the proper development of nerve cells and red blood cells and helps prevent anemia while helping metabolize protein, carbohydrates, fat, and homocysteine levels in the blood. Cyanocobalamin is a lab-made version of this vitamin that has shown to be effective via pill and injection. In addition, the following foods are good sources of B12: Yogurt, grass-fed beef and cow's milk, lamb, shellfish, salmon, sardines, and scallops.

Vitamin C (ascorbic acid) works as an antioxidant to counter free radicals and is also necessary for the production of serotonin. It strengthens blood vessels, protects the body from bacterial toxins, helps metabolize tyrosine and tryptophan, and works as an antihistamine.

Vitamin D3 is a fat-soluble vitamin that promotes calcium absorption and enables normal mineralization and growth of the bones. Deficiency of Vitamin D3 (the active source of Vitamin D) can lead to loss of bone density, brittle bones or misshapen bones. Ample levels can help prevent osteoporosis. Studies show that those with the lowest serum vitamin D levels have a two-fold risk of chronic headaches over those with the highest levels. It is important that you ask your healthcare provider to test your Vitamin D blood levels to ensure you do not get too much.

Vitamin E is a fat-soluble vitamin with strong anti-oxidant properties. It protects pituitary, adrenal and sex hormones, and increases the rate at which new blood vessels develop around damaged areas while helping to normalize blood viscosity. The most important components of Vitamin E appear to be the tocopherols. All four forms of tocopherol have been shown to have antioxidant activity, but alpha-tocopherol is the strongest antioxidant. Alpha-tocopherol inhibits the oxidation of LDL, which can help prevent LDL from sticking to the arterial walls. In addition to its antioxidant properties, vitamin E also acts to reduce blood coagulation and may help lower blood pressure by eliciting endothelial relaxation.

Vitamin K2 helps prevent osteoporosis by keeping calcium in your bones where it belongs. Without vitamin K2, calcium floats through your bloodstream and sticks to places it doesn't belong, like your blood vessels.

IONIC MINERALS

The human body is a miracle of electrical impulses that keep it functioning and make life possible. Ionic minerals are an essential part in this process, as the body relies on them to conduct and generate electrical impulses. Without the correct balance on ionic minerals in the body, your brain and muscles could not function properly and cells could not properly absorb nutrients.

There are over 70 trace minerals that are important to cellular, neurologic, joint, and bone health. Taken together, ionic minerals balance and replace electrolytes, maintain pH balance, improve circulatory health, and aid absorption of vitamins and nutrients.

Since most people do not live by the sea and much of our soil is depleted of minerals, many are deficient in these essential elements. Taking supplements containing ionic minerals can help arthritis in many ways, as long as the minerals are produced in water soluble form. A few of the most important ionic minerals are the following:

Boron: Helps metabolize calcium and magnesium and is critical for healthy membrane function

Calcium: Important for healthy teeth and bones, and helps regulate nerve function

Chromium: Stimulates enzymes involved in glucose metabolism, increases effectiveness of insulin, and stimulates the synthesis of fatty acids

Copper: Essential for healthy function of proteins and enzymes, and aids in the absorption of iron

Iron: Needed to transport oxygen to the cells in your body.

Magnesium: Plays important roles in a wide array of physiological processes. It is absorbed in the gastrointestinal tract and helps facilitate the absorption of calcium. In addition to pill and powder supplements, magnesium is naturally found in foods like seeds (sesame, sunflower), nuts (cashews, almonds), spices, meat, dairy products, green leafy vegetables (Swiss chard, spinach), tea, coffee, cocoa, black beans, and halibut. Your body needs a certain amount every day; if you take too much, you will experience diarrhea.

Manganese: Promotes healthy bone formation, supports growth of healthy connective tissue, and boosts calcium absorption.

Phosphorous: Helps repair damaged cells and promotes healthy new cell growth

Potassium: Stimulates nerve impulses, acts with sodium to regulate fluids and stimulate the kidneys, and helps convert glucose to glycogen.

Selenium: A powerful antioxidant that helps Vitamin E protect cells and connective tissue by destroying free radicals. Selenium is an important antioxidant for chemical detoxification.

Zinc: Helps boost white blood cell production in your immune system. Zinc is necessary for absorption of the B-complex vitamins. It is a component of insulin, and a constituent of over 25 enzymes involved in digestion and metabolism.

PROTEOLYTIC ENZYMES

For headache and migraine relief, it is important to have proteolytic activity on the systemic level. Known as protease, this category of enzymes acts as a catalyst in the breakdown of proteins into peptides or amino acids. This helps control both systemic inflammation. Proteolytic enzymes also provide essential antioxidant and cardiovascular support. I will discuss two of the more potent ones next.

Bromelian is a mix of proteolytic enzymes (those found in pineapples), which have been used for centuries to help indigestion and reduce inflammation. Studies indicate this product helps reduce pain, especially when used in combination with some other natural pain-relieving agents.

Papain contains a wide array of proteolytic enzymes, incorporating a broad range of substrate specificity and optimum environments. Because of this attribute, Papain easily and efficiently hydrolyzes most soluble protein, yielding peptides, and amino acids. Papain has an effective pH range of 3.0 to 10.5.

HOW TO TAKE NATURAL SUPPLEMENTS

Because natural supplements are made of organically existing substances, they affect the body in gentle ways — without side effects. The ingredients within natural supplements often do not work as quickly as drugs do at relieving pain or inflammation. However, they do offer acute relief in the short term while working more powerfully over time to create a gradual and lasting change in condition. In other words, supplements need to build up in your system to get to a level where more significant change occurs, which is why you often will need to take them several times per day, over periods of weeks and months or even longer.

The best way to take supplements is by following the guidelines on the label. These guidelines are often the minimal doses, and, for acute conditions, the doses can be increased, sometimes doubled or tripled. However, in high doses even natural substances can become toxic in the body. In all cases, it is necessary to use caution and to take supplements and medications as directed on the bottle or as suggested by a professional healthcare provider.

CHAPTER REVIEW

- Natural supplements are far superior to chemically manufactured medicines for gently re-balancing the body to help reduce and prevent headaches and migraines.

- When taken as directed, natural ingredients in supplements are less toxic to the body, and can reduce pain and inflammation without side effects

- Natural supplements affect the body in gentle ways, and require more time to build up in the body to make a positive change

- Certain supplements provide vitamins and minerals that are difficult or nearly impossible for us to get naturally; yet, understanding the source of them is crucial to health

- Supplements with some of the following ingredients are critical to relieve pain and inflammation associated with headaches: Boswella extract, burdock root, butterbur, feverfew, omega-3 fatty acids, rutin, SAMe, curcumin, white willow bark, kudzu, lavender, lemongrass, and many others outlines in the chapter.

- When taking supplements, always follow the guidelines on the label and discuss dosing with your health care provider

CHAPTER 11

STRESS REDUCTION AND MEDITATION FOR HEADACHE RELIEF

Stress is one of the leading causes of illness in the United States. Nearly 66% or two-thirds of all signs and symptoms presented in doctors' offices in the U.S. are stress related. Most people who suffer chronic headaches and migraine also suffer the ill effects of stress. The inability to do what they used to be able to do, coupled with pain and inflammation, creates physical, psychological, and emotional stress.

THE NASTY EFFECTS OF STRESS

As briefly discussed earlier, the effects of stress include nail biting, anxiety, a racing mind, obsessive thoughts, compulsive behavior, unending worry, muscle tension and spasm, poor or too great an appetite, digestive disorders, constipation, insomnia, poor blood flow, belabored breathing, neck pain, shoulder tension, and the possible onset or continuation of bad habits such as dependence on alcohol, drugs, painkillers, food, and caffeine.

Any one of these things by itself can trigger a number of different types of headache. But when these forces of antagonism are combined (as they generally are when triggered by stress), the headache problems often become chronic and insufferable. In short, stress makes headaches worse and headaches cause more stress. It's a vicious cycle that needs to be broken. Before I show you how, let's look at the psychology of stress to better understand the solutions presented.

THE PSYCHOLOGY OF STRESS

Stress is an interesting phenomenon. It means different things to different people. What we each individually consider to be stressful is largely a matter of our perception. Our perceptions are our realities and so what we think is posing a threat is actually doing so by virtue of our established belief system. Moreover, there are many kinds of stressors – physical (the response to being frightened), emotional (loss of a loved one), psychological (obsessive thoughts), spiritual (loss of faith), and psychosomatic (the need for attention).

Physiologically, stress is responsible for initiating the fight-or-flight response in the face of perceived danger. This means when we are confronted by danger, our body automatically prepares us to deal with the coming stressful situation by focusing our attention, pumping more blood into our muscles, and sending adrenaline through our system to ready it for action. It is precisely this response that helps protect the body and return it again to homeostasis. However, too much stress, or stress left unresolved for too long a time, can lead to biological damage.

You see, at the onset of perceived danger, the body is quickly jolted into fight-or-flight mode, which means stress hormones such as adrenaline and cortisol are pumped into the bloodstream.

However, at the conclusion of the danger episode, the body does not automatically calm down and return to homeostasis. In fact, it takes a great deal of time for the body to return to so-called normal conditions. But often this cannot happen because another stressor may present itself (e.g., sitting in traffic, standing in line at the bank, missing a deadline), and this sends our body into "code red" mode all over again.

The effects of such prolonged or recurring stress is that it keeps the autonomic nervous system from balancing, which can lead to problems with the gastrointestinal tract, the digestive system, the respiratory system, and the neuroendocrine system. "The Headache Relief Action Plan" offers many solutions for each aspect of the headache and migraine puzzle. In terms of stress reduction, the plan includes a mind-body approach for long-term success. In the short term, there are simpler solutions to bust the stress as it arises. Here are 10 solutions.

10 SIMPLE STRESS BUSTERS

The idea behind living stress-free is to remove the things in your life that cause you to be stressed. Of course, this is easier said than done, but it is truly the only way to not have stress. Here are 10 simple things you can do daily to reduce the symptoms of stress.

1. Walk outside for at least 20 continuous minutes every day.
2. Quiet the mind and calm the nerves with meditation.
3. Take 10 deep belly breaths every hour.
4. Drink plenty of pure water – at least 10 glasses a day.
5. Avoid sugar and caffeine in all forms.

6. Regulate sleep and wake cycles to a consistent daily routine.
7. Prioritize your life, work, family, and personal time and activities.
8. Do six shoulder shrugs whenever you are tense.
9. Realize that when people criticize and judge, they are labeling an "image" of you and not you personally.
10. Realize that you are worth so much more than the sum of your titles, money, and belongings.

A good stress-relief program should be followed when controlling headaches. Good programs generally include various forms of meditation. Stress is a monster that really takes its toll. Let's look at how relaxation and meditation can reduce your stress and also change your genes.

CENTERING MIND AND EMOTIONS

Since the mind controls and constructs perceptions and the emotions act and react toward threatening stimuli, the daily centering of the mind and emotions is essential to headache prevention. While there are many method of centering the mind and emotions, meditation is one of the most powerful and convenient techniques we have.

In Mosby's *Complementary and Alternative Medicine*, Freeman and Lawlis include, among a list of areas where meditation is successful as a medical intervention, the following known headache triggers and symptoms: chronic pain, gastrointestinal distress, headache, anxiety and panic, sleep disturbances, job and family stress, Type A behavior, and panic disorders.[1]

The large-scale integration of meditation into medical setting happened in Boston, largely through the tireless efforts of Herbert

Benson, MD. After researching meditation techniques across many cultures, with a specific focus on the Transcendental Meditation of Maharishi Mahash Yogi, Dr. Benson came to develop what is known simply as the "Relaxation Response."

THE RELAXATION RESPONSE

Decades ago, Dr. Benson participated in conversations between scientists and Buddhists that were initiated by the 14th Dalai Lama. These discussions were organized by the Mind & Life Institute.

According to Benson, the relaxation response is "a physical state of deep rest that changes the physical and emotional responses to stress... and the opposite of the fight-or-flight response." The fight-or-flight response, an elevated state of excitation that causes harm in the body when it goes on too long, can be reduced or countered by meditation.

Benson proved that practicing meditative techniques to induce the relaxation response creates a healthier environment within the body. Heart rate, breath rate, blood pressure, and body pain are all reduced through this type of relaxation. But Benson also investigated if the meditative state of deep relaxation had prolonged effects on human biology that were not merely temporary. This has intriguing implications for the vascular and neurological nature of headaches and migraines.

Benson's method is clear and easy to do, and it is concerned only with the relaxation response (not spiritual enlightenment or other transpersonal goals). It consists of two parts:

Part 1: For 10 to 20 minutes, continuously repeat a word, phrase, sound, prayer or movement and align it with your natural breathing cycle.

Part 2 When outside noises or thoughts intrude during practice, simply take notice of them and avoid judgment or response to them. Simply return to the task at hand.

These two parts are the basic guidelines. There are nine steps to the actual practice that help create a deep state of relaxation when the relaxation response can be induced. Benson's relaxation response consists of the following steps:

1. Choose the focus of your meditation (a single word, prayer, movement, etc.).
2. Lie down or sit still in a comfortable position.
3. Close your eyes.
4. Relax your muscles. (This can be done progressively, scanning from the toes to the tip of the head.)
5. Focus on your breathing. (Observe your breath as it moves in and out of your body, without stressing over it.)
6. Silently repeat the chosen word or prayer or do the selected motion with each exhalation.
7. Repeat this process of focusing on your breath while repeating the word or movement for 10 to 20 minutes.
8. After completion, sit quietly for a few moments, eyes closed, to reawaken into the world.
9. Do not stress about or over think how well you are meditating or able to hold the phrase or observe the breath. Just allow it to happen.

MINDFULNESS AND HEADACHES

One of the most studied and popular meditation methods in the world is called Mindfulness. Several journals have reported on the effectiveness of mindfulness meditation on migraine and tension-type headaches in particular.

The journal *Headache* reported on a study carried out by researchers at Wake Forest Baptist Medical Center.[3] They looked to assess the safety, feasibility, and effects of the standardized 8-week mindfulness-based stress reduction (MBSR) course in adults with migraines. At the end of the 8-week period, the MBSR participants had 1.4 fewer migraines per month than the control group who received "usual care" for their migraines. While pain did decrease slightly more than the control group's reported pain, MBSR participants had migraines that were on average 2.9 hours shorter in duration.

"We found that the MBSR participants had trends of fewer migraines that were less severe," says Rebecca Erwin Wells, an assistant professor of neurology at Wake Forest Baptist Medical Center. "Secondary effects included headaches that were shorter in duration and less disabling, and participants had increases in mindfulness and self-efficacy—a sense of personal control over their migraines. In addition, there were no adverse events and excellent adherence." The *International Journal of Psychophysiology* reported on a randomized, controlled experiment that found those suffering migraine and tension-type headaches had increased heart rate variability (HRV; variation in time interval between heart beats) while engaging in mindfulness after a stressful encounter. The researchers concluded:

> *"Associations between headache conditions (migraine, tension) and imbalances in the autonomic nervous system (ANS) are due to stress-related dysregulation in the activity*

of the parasympathetic-sympathetic branches. Mindfulness meditation has demonstrated effectiveness in reducing pain-related distress, and in enhancing heart rate variability—a vagal-mediated marker of ANS balance. This study examined HRV during cognitive stress and mindfulness meditation in individuals with migraine and tension headaches."[4]

MEDITATION REQUIRES GRADUAL PROGRESS

In the beginning stages of learning to meditate, you may experience the following things: a tendency to fall asleep; the mind appears to race more than usual, which it probably isn't, but your senses are heightened and you are noticing it more fully; your legs will begin to fall asleep or tingle from poor flexibility or cramping; and, you unknowingly lose focus of your breathing and find that your mind has wandered to another part of your body or to a drifting thought. All of this is okay and normal.

Like anything else, progress is made slowly and gradually over time. It is advised to practice this meditative exercise twice per day: In the early morning, and in the late evening before bed. In this way, you relax at night for optimal repair and wake refreshed and ready to start the day in the best state possible. Continue the daily practice for an extended period of time (months and even years), and the results you experience may be life changing.

While many like to meditate first thing in the morning to begin the day at a level place, I like to meditate before going to sleep. This way, I have uninterrupted time and nothing pressing to keep my mind alert for after the session. And once the relaxation response is activated, I allow myself to drift off into a deep and restful sleep, where healing occurs.

Whether you do it in the morning or evening, getting restful sleep is essential to physical repair and stress reduction. In fact, when you sleep, your body metabolizes the harmful stress hormones that cause pain and weight gain. In the next chapter, we'll look at how improper sleeping can cause you additional pain and how correct sleeping can improve your quality of life and help you overcome headaches and migraines.

CHAPTER REVIEW

- Stress is a leading causes of illness in the United States, accounting for almost 66% of doctors' office visits.
- The effects of stress are numerous; while it's a natural response, an excess of stress will lead to biological damage.
- Prolonged or recurring stress keeps the autonomic nervous system from balancing, which can lead to problems with the gastrointestinal tract, the digestive system, the respiratory system, and the neuroendocrine system. It breaks down the body's immune system, and causes inflammation and negative changes to the neurological and vascular systems.
- Stress can also lead to depression, anxiety, muscle tension, insomnia, and body pain. All of these are known triggers of various mental and physical (mind-body) illnesses and diseases, including headaches and migraines.
- Review the "10 Simple Stress Busters" again and often.
- You can derail the negative effects of stress by inducing deep mental and physical relaxation through daily meditation and mindfulness practices.

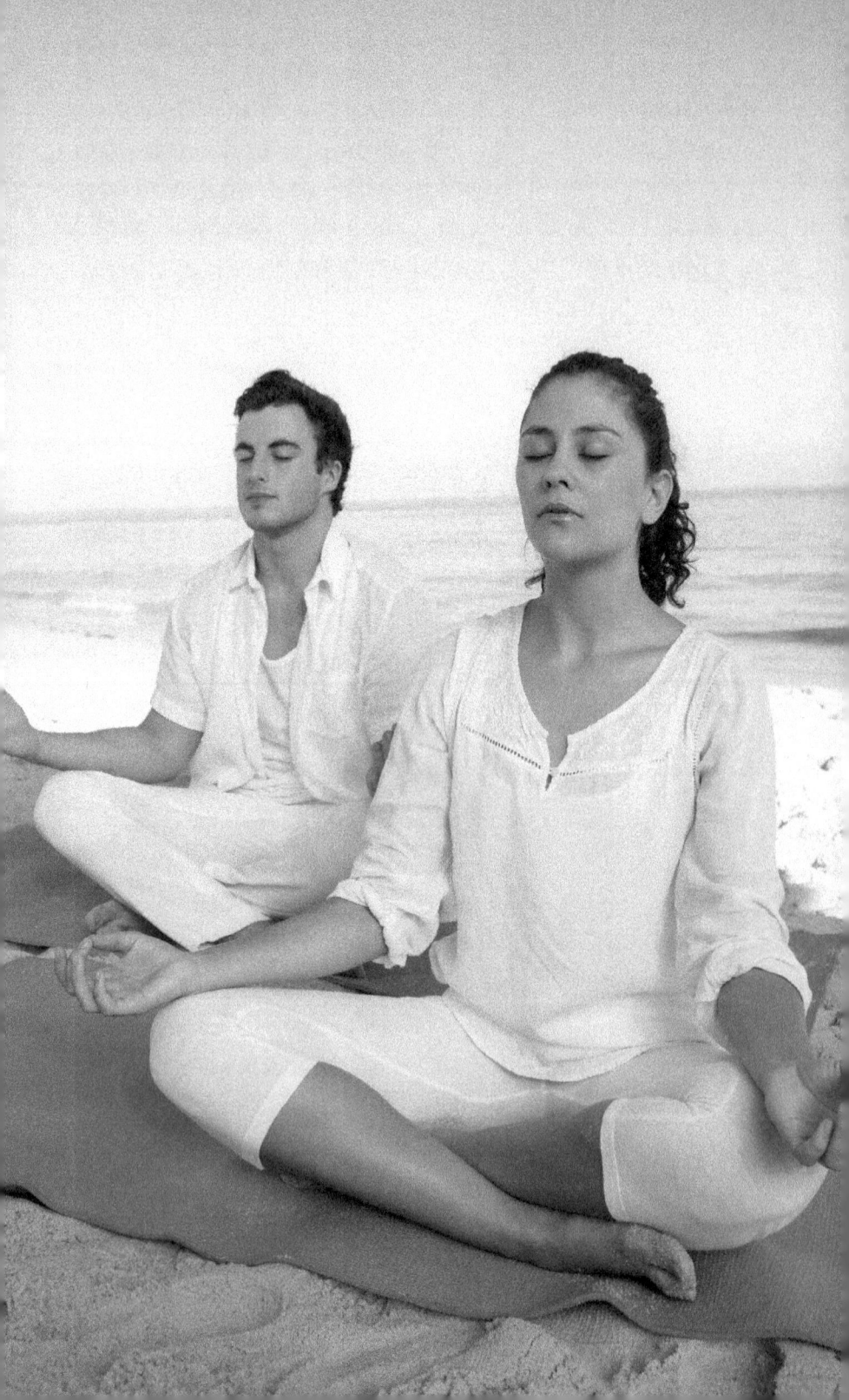

CHAPTER 12

BREATHING EXERCISES FOR HEADACHE RELIEF

Mild oxygen deprivation causes headaches and generalized chronic pain. Caused by poor breathing patterns or breathing obstruction, this is one of the hidden, yet most direct and preventable headache triggers. Life begins with a breath and a cry and ends with a final exhalation. Yet, while the atmosphere offers us an ample oxygen supply, we neglect to put it to best use. We rarely fill our lungs. We take quick short breaths and compromise our health.

The Chinese have a proverb that loosely translates as:

When you're born, you intuitively inhale deeply from your stomach;
at middle age, you breathe from the middle of your chest;
as you approach the end of life, your breath is restricted to your throat.

Proper breathing allows many vital life functions to occur, including filling the body with ample levels of oxygen to feed the blood and brain, to burn food and release energy, and to expel toxic carbon monoxide with each exhale. In other words, the less full and more superficial our breathing, the closer to death we seem to be. We should breathe from our stomachs, expanding and contracting the abdomen, which facilitates a full and complete breathing cycle. It draws fresh air to the bottom of the lungs and expels stale air from the same depths.

MILD OXYGEN DEPRIVATION CAUSES HEADACHES

Though we don't consciously think of it, the way we breathe has a direct effect on our state of health and well-being, with the power to make us ill or to heal us. Have you ever been so scared you forgot to breathe, when, for example, a car suddenly pulled out in front of you? How about the last time you were feeling stressed out? If you were too busy or preoccupied to do something about it, your breath became short and belabored, and this perhaps led to you getting a dull, pounding headache. If you took a moment to draw in a few deep breaths, you could have become instantly more relaxed and your breathing cycle would have become steady, thus averting the headache.

YAWNING AND SNORING

Yawning is a sure sign that our bodies are lacking in oxygen, as the process brings in a deep breath of air in one instant. Shallow breathing occurs when you are tired, under stress or have been sitting still for a long time. Not only is yawning a sure sign that our bodies are in need of more oxygen, it can also be a sign that an oxygen-deprivation headache may be on its way.

Without an ample supply of fresh oxygen in the lungs, cells, tissues, and organs will be unable to function properly. When this happens, the levels of toxins and histamines in the bloodstream increases causing vascular headaches, such as migraine and cluster. What happens is the blood vessels have to widen to allow more oxygen-carrying blood to flow through them. This vasodilation is the cause of headache pain. The easiest way to prevent this from happening is by increasing physical activity and engaging in simple breathing exercises.

People who either snore when they sleep, sleep with their head face-down on their pillow, or sleep in areas where there is poor ventilation, are susceptible to getting cluster headaches. In these cases, the cluster headache is the result of low levels of oxygen in the blood and brain due to an obstruction in the nasal passages. At the advice and prescription of their doctors, some sufferers of oxygen-deprivation headaches find great relief with a CPAP machine or oxygen tank.

There are two main types of oxygen therapy: oxidation and oxygenation. Both of these treatments have been proven effective in treating conditions such as circulatory problems, chronic fatigue syndrome, allergies, and headaches.[1] In fact, studies show that keeping a tank of pure oxygen by their beds and inhaling the air through a mask works to abort a cluster headache in progress. Inhaling pure oxygen has been clinically proven to decrease cluster headaches by as much as 80%.[2] While oxygen therapy may provide instant relief, which is terrific, it will not correct improper breathing throughout the day and night from triggering headaches again and again.

Proper and sufficient intake of oxygen requires only that you breathe in the proper way, and that you practice deep breathing techniques when stress and tension begin to take hold in your body. These, of course, lead to slower blood flow and oxygen-deprivation headaches. Deep breathing increases levels of oxygen in the lungs, enhances respiratory functions and oxygen levels in the blood, and improves delivery of oxygen to the cells. Moreover, the taking of continuous full breaths allows for more oxygen to reach the head and nourish the central nervous system. "The Headache Relief Action Plan" includes a set of breathing exercises that are easy to learn and do, don't take much time, and help prevent and stop headaches of this nature in their tracks.

6 TIPS FOR BETTER BREATHING

TIP 1 - Keep your work, social, and sleep areas well ventilated.

TIP 2 - Sleep on a pillow that is not too fluffy, and don't let it cover your nose when you sleep.

TIP 3 - Sleep on your back or side.

TIP 4 - Use sinus strips to prevent obstructed breathing while sleeping.

TIP 5 - Make it a habit to take about a dozen slow, deep breaths each hour or as often as possible.

TIP 6 - Eat a mucus-free diet (avoid dairy, wheat and processed foods) to reduce phlegm.

HEADACHE-BUSTING BREATHING EXERCISES

Deep breathing practices have been embraced by Eastern mystics and healers for thousands of years, as evidenced in breathwork's major standing in yoga and Qigong practices. In fact, a study on deep breathing in India revealed that after 15 minutes of practice, the average volume of air taken into the lungs on inhalation rose from 482 ml before practice to 740 ml afterward, while the average number of breaths per minute dropped from 15 down to five. This represents a huge improvement in respiratory efficiency.[3]

Breathing exercises increase overall oxygen consumption in the lungs and flow through the blood and to the brain which positively reduces the onset of headaches with psychosomatic triggers (like stress and anxiety) and should be performed upon waking from a breath-obstructed sleep. Deep breathing has the power to alter consciousness, calm the mind, center the spirit, and relax tense muscles. Once you experience the feeling of deep breathing, you will be able to do it at any time your body may queue you to do so—such as when tensions seize your shoulders and spine, when your breath becomes shallow from stress and anxiety due to deadline-driven workloads or by a dull, pounding headache caused by shallow breathing.

To reap the full benefits of breathing as a means of preventing headache triggers and reducing their symptoms of pain, nausea, and shortness of breath, the following exercises should be performed once time per day at a minimum, and more often as needed during high stress times.

ABDOMINAL BREATHING EXERCISE

1. Lie down on your back, with knees bent and feet placed flat on the floor a foot's distance from your buttocks.
2. Make sure your lower back is resting on the floor and not arched.
3. Inhale deeply by allowing your abdomen to rise (expand) as you inhale to fill your lungs to capacity.

4. Allow your abdomen to sink (contract) on exhale to fully expel all of the air (fresh and stale) from the lower quadrants of your lungs.
5. Repeat this no less than a dozen times during each cycle.
6. Try to be *mindful* of the experience as a whole while engaging in it.

CHEST BREATHING EXERCISE

1. Stand in a comfortable position with shoulders relaxed, hands by your sides, and legs shoulder's width apart.
2. Close your eyes and make sure your neck, shoulders, arms, and legs are relaxed.
3. Inhale through your nose evenly and quietly, pulling oxygen into your lungs, expanding them to full capacity. Be sure to inflate the chest only, not the stomach.
4. Exhale slightly longer than the inhalation, and, as you do, push the stale breath out through your mouth slowly, evenly and quietly. Be sure to contract your chest and lungs to their least capacity.
5. You may perform this exercise as often as you like throughout the day, but not for more than five minutes at any one time.

CHAPTER REVIEW

- Chronic, mild oxygen deprivation is one of the most common, and most preventable, triggers of headache and migraine.
- Taking and maintaining steady, full breaths are essential for reducing the stress response, regulating the nervous system, and reducing and preventing headaches.
- Incorporate the six tips for better breathing to help reduce this trigger.
- When you feel a headache coming on or notice your breathing is belabored, do one or both of the breathing exercises described in this chapter.

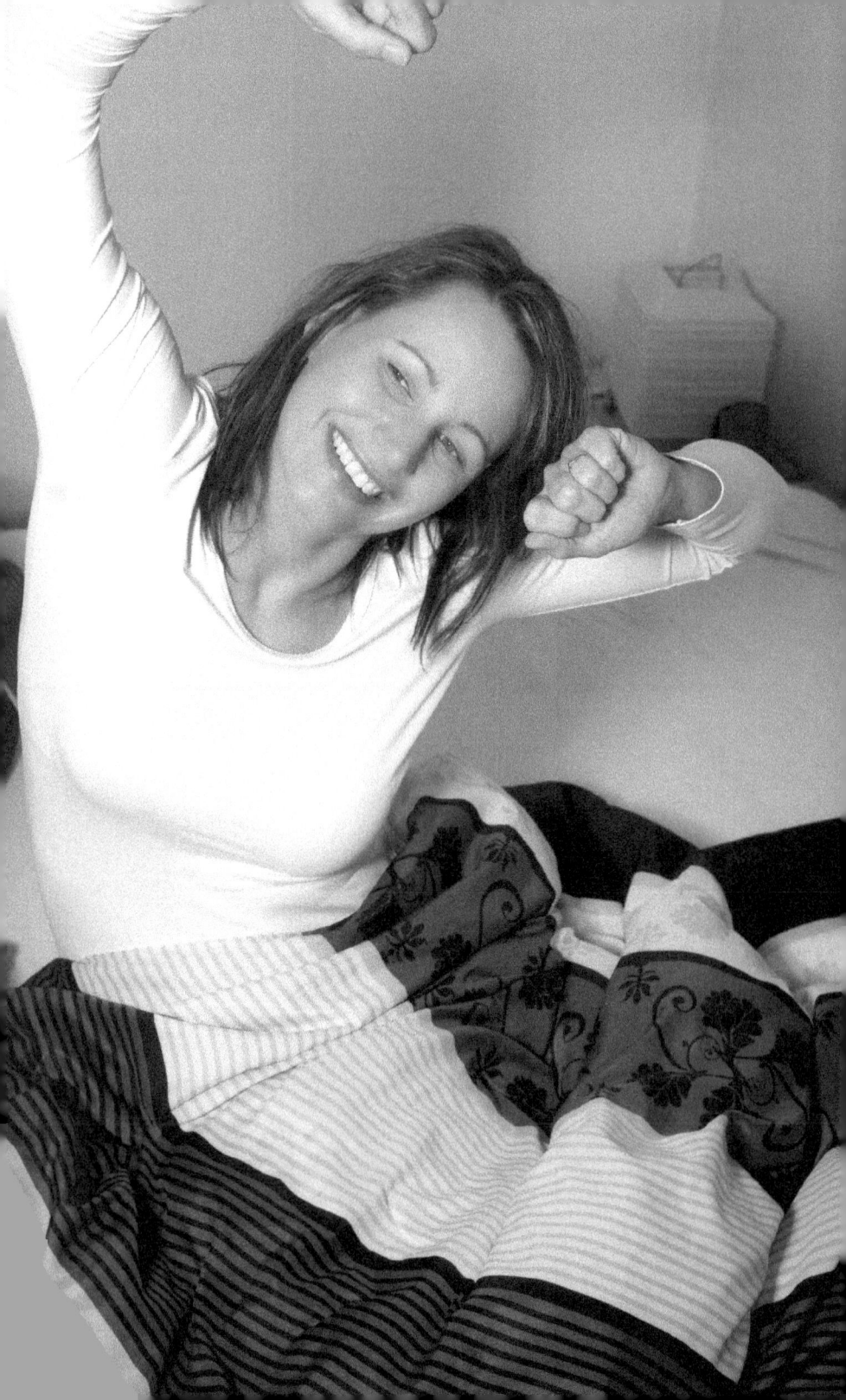

CHAPTER 13

SLEEP YOUR WAY TO HEADACHE RELIEF

Mathematically speaking, the average person spends nearly one-third of their life asleep—or at least in bed. However, statistics show that sleep disorders are among the nation's most common health problems, affecting up to 70 million people.[1] For those suffering chronic headaches, sleep is often something they get too much or too little. Either way, when at either extreme, it's a bad thing.

Sleep deprivation is a sure trigger of headaches. Anxiety, stress, digestive issues, consuming alcohol at night, and low levels of serotonin lead to poor sleeping patterns. Proper, sound sleep happens in distinct stages, and these stages regulate the deep tissue healing of our muscles, relax the nervous systems, and regulate hormones and help reestablish homeostasis.

Improper restorative rest after exercise or long weeks of stress-laden work, and general insomnia or the inability to sleep straight through the night do much to trigger both migraine headaches and muscle-contraction (tension-type) headaches. If you do get a sound sleep but also experience headaches on waking, it may be caused by either lack of oxygen to the brain or from poor sleep posture, which puts pressure on nerves and stunts blood flow in the body during the evening hours.

Getting a sound sleep and doing so in a posture that will neither cramp the muscles nor constrict air supply is vital to preventing headaches. The best position to sleep in is lying on your back with arms by your sides, and head and neck straight and slightly elevated. Another good posture is the fetal position, as long as the arms are kept in front of the body and not shoved under the pillow or raised above the head. There are several ergonomic pillows available today that make finding a comfortable yet proper sleeping posture easy.

As a person who suffered from excruciating headaches and musculoskeletal pain for over 30 years, let me assure you that sound sleep is a wonder boon nobody can do without. Both the sleep-deprivation and poor sleep posture headache triggers are totally correctable and preventable!

REGULAR, SOUND SLEEP IS ESSENTIAL

Sleep is not only a fundamental human need, it is a necessity that no one who experiences aches or pains of any kind should ever take for granted. It is so important that our bodies tell our brains when certain essential chemicals have been depleted and our muscles and ligaments are tired and in need of restoration.

The growing problem is that many of us rely on legal stimulants such as coffee, tea, and sodas, to force ourselves to continue plugging away. After all, work cannot be held back by pleading there are just not enough hours in the week. The result? We stay up too late, we get up too early, and to do this, we consume unhealthy amounts of toxic substances—night after night after night… and all day, too.

The net result? For the better part of our adult lives, we and our coworkers are both sick AND tired; and it is constantly taking its toll. Let's look at some of the damage we've done to ourselves by simply not going to sleep when we are tired.

In our natural circadian rhythm or biological clock, sleep is set to take over during the evening hours. We are genetically programmed to get up and lie down with the sun. So it was with the invention of artificial sources of light (candles and bulbs) that our stressed-out drive for more working hours at the expense of much-needed rest began.

What's the big deal, you ask, if you sleep only a few hours per night? You can always drink coffee, take No-Doze caffeine pills, cat naps… life is good. Well, not really. Did you know that in clinical tests, rats die within a few short weeks of sleep deprivation? And it's not just the lab rats at risk; it's people like me and you that are at risk, too.

Chronic fatigue, adrenal fatigue, attention deficit disorder, chronic migraines and headaches, body aches and pain, mental illness, depression, and anxiety are all in part caused—or made worse—by lack of sleep. And no caffeine pill or taurine-laced energy drink can cure these dangerous side-effects of our global-economy-size workloads.

Exercising at night is also a problem for those prone to insomnia. If you exercise between dinner and bedtime, change your workout schedule. It's keeping you up by moving blood and energy through your system. Researchers at Stanford University School of Medicine found that adults ages 55 to 75 who engaged in 20 to 30 minutes of low-impact exercise (like walking) every other day in the afternoon fell asleep in half the average, normal time. What's more, their sleep duration increased on average by one full hour.

EIGHT TIPS FOR A RESTFUL NIGHT'S SLEEP

So you say for you, it isn't a crazy work schedule? You just have trouble drifting off and staying asleep? Here are eight tips to help you overcome insomnia:

TIP 1 - Do not consume ANY sugar or caffeine after 6:00pm.

TIP 2 - Stop working at least two hours before bedtime.

TIP 3 - Turn off the computer and television at least one hour before bedtime.

TIP 4 - Make sure your sleeping quarters are as dark and silent as possible. Studies have shown that those in darker and quieter spaces tend to sleep through the night more deeply than others.

TIP 5 - Establish a standard sleep/wake schedule, and stick to it.

TIP 6 - Place a notepad next to your bed and when your mind starts racing with things that need to get done, or people that need to be called, simply write it down and *let it go* until the morning. Lying awake in bed at night will in no way help these things get done; it only amplifies stress and anxiety and prevents sleep.

TIP 7 - Make a set routine out of bedtime. Change into pajamas, brush your teeth, set out clothes for the morning, even jot down any last thoughts, but promise yourself to revisit them tomorrow, and then turn off the light… breathe deeply, relax, sleep tight.

TIP 8 - If a racing mind is nagging, do the progressive relaxation technique taught below. It will induce a deep state of calm and relaxation that should allow you to drift off to sleep in short time while allowing your body and nervous system to rejuvenate.

PROGRESSIVE RELAXATION TECHNIQUE

Progressive relaxation induces such a deep state of relaxation that most people fall asleep before reaching the arm portion of this exercise. Give it a try and see how it goes. And if you find it difficult at first, don't stress out—it's only a relaxation technique. Let your thoughts go and enjoy the process and perhaps sooner than later it will take hold and you will begin enjoying the deep full sleep that may have been missing from their life for many years.

1. Lie on your back with arms at your sides and slowly inhale and exhale with no sound.

2. Do cyclical breathing, with a four-second count for a full inhalation and an eight-second count for a full exhalation. Do a count of at least 10 repetitions, but more if necessary.

3. Once your respiration is calm and even, return to normal breathing and begin progressively relaxing every part of your body by mentally focusing on that area, calmly willing it to relax and retaining your intention there until the part begins to tingle.

4. Begin by relaxing the toes of the left leg, one at a time. Then move on to the sole of the foot, the ankle, the calf and so on until you reach the hips. Then do the same with the right leg.

5. Move progressively up to the buttocks, hips, back, arms, chest, shoulders, neck, and face.

WRONG SLEEPING CAUSES PAIN

The power of restorative rest and sleep is strong and wide reaching. But did you know that improper sleep can be a cause of pain and suffering? Poor sleeping posture is the reason for this. While there are many ways to sleep and many products that allow us to sleep in those ways, there are actually only two healthy positions for engaging in sound slumber. Before we look at those, let's review some of the more common sleeping positions and why they are harmful to the body.

Stomach Sleeping

Stomach sleepers, well, sleep on their stomachs. Usually they have one or both arms extended over their heads, their face turned either to the left or right side and one leg is generally bent.

There are so many problems with this posture. First, sleeping with the arms extended over the head raises the shoulders into the neck, causing cramping, poor circulation and pain. It also skews the trapezius muscles and skeletal system, compressing the thoracic outlet where the brachial plexus of nerves from the neck travel down the arms to the hands.

Second, when the arms are raised the nerves are irritated and nerve function is either inhibited or excited. It's a neurological and vascular response that affects the brachial plexus of nerves that travels from the neck and down the arms. The effect is tingling and/or numbness in the arms or hands. Ever wake up with pins and needles in the hands or a "dead" arm? This may be why.

Third, sleeping with the neck turned to one side creates unbalanced muscles, where one side is hypertonic (contracted) and the other is hypotonic (extended). This leads to neck strain, cramping, pain, and often headaches.

Fourth, the bent leg stretches one leg and hip all night, while the other remains prone. Again, this imbalance can lead to hip and leg pain.

And fifth, stomach sleeping offers too little support for the abdomen, allowing the stomach to fall forward and the lumbar region of the back to sag. This can make your gut seem bigger than it is, simply because of poor sleeping posture. It also creates spinal compression and lower back pain. By extension, there can be cervical irritation and spasm in the neck causing headaches.

Comfortable or not, this position has to be avoided if you want restful, sound sleep that does not place your body in a way that triggers muscle-contraction or oxygen-deprivation headaches.

Back Sleeping

Back sleepers are on to something. The back is one of the two best ways to sleep because it can offer solid support for your entire musculoskeletal system.

Problems arise for back sleepers, however, when they do not place pillows under their knees. If you are lying on your back and your legs are straight, there is insufficient support for the lower back allowing it to arch too high.

If you sleep on your back with one leg bent, you probably experience the same hip, lower back and/or knee strain and pain as do the stomach sleepers who sleep in this way.

You should always place two pillows under your knees for support and one pillow under your head. Keep in mind, too, that pillows are for sleeping support, not just for comfort. Your head should be placed squarely on your pillow, and the pillow should be pulled down enough so that it touches your shoulders. If your pillow is not touching your shoulders, you run the risk of not supporting the cervical vertebrae and neck muscles, resulting in pain that results from spasm or nerve impingement.

Side Sleeping

Side sleeping gets my vote for best sleeping position, if done correctly. To begin, side posture should mimic the fetal position. That is, both knees bent with hands held close to the body. This is a normal and inherent sleeping posture.

Errors in side sleeping occur when one leg overlaps the other. This causes an imbalance in the hips that can lead to tightness and pain in the hip flexors, IT band, low back, and knees.

Another common error is sleeping with hands under or over the head and scrunching the pillow so your head is elevated. Symptoms from this can include neck and shoulder pain, stiffness, headaches, and tingling or numbness in the arms or hands.

Side sleeping is the best because it allows the body to maintain a proper and corrective posture for several hours. What you should do is place a pillow between your knees to create proper distance between them, which keeps the hips in proper balance. The legs must be parallel so the hips remain square and there is no strain on the low back. A pillow should be placed under the head and pulled to the shoulder for optimal neck support. The hands should be parallel and below the eyes.

Who knew there was so much to sleeping posture? Try these corrections, then after a while your daily neck strain, shoulder pain, headaches, hip and low back pain, and arm tingling may just start to correct itself.

DON'T SLEEP ON NEGATIVE FEELINGS

Difficult decisions can be made easier by "sleeping on it." However, the opposite is true for unfortunate news, trauma, a big argument or any emotional upset, as sleep makes your bad feelings worse. So reduce mental strain after unpleasantness by staying awake for a while even if it's the middle of the night. Otherwise, giving in to sleep magnifies and promotes your unsettled feelings. As we will see in Chapter 14, the mind-body connection is very real and emotions are often trapped in the body—becoming a "pain body"— and trigger chronic migraines, cluster headaches, tension headaches, and pain in general.

A recent study by researchers at the University of Massachusetts (Amherst), and published in the *Journal of Neuroscience*, found that sleeping too soon after a traumatic event locks in bad memories and emotions.[2] This is an important concept; extended time spent in a poor emotional state is not healthy. Too much sadness can lead to depression. Too much crying impacts the lungs, which helps regulate oxygen in the body. Wallowing in bad memories and reflecting on hard or emotional times brings those moments into the present and makes you live them all over again. It also impairs your feelings, your emotions, and your energy in the present. Repeatedly reliving negative experiences is virtually the same as having those experiences over again and again in the present. Negative memories and emotions trigger one another and set the body into a frequency of unhealthy energy.

The Amherst researchers found that you don't even have to experience an actual, negative event to suffer. Merely seeing troubling images in your mind is enough to cause lasting emotional trauma… if you sleep on it. University of Massachusetts neuroscientist Rebecca Spencer, one of the study's co-authors said, "Not only did sleep protect the memory, but it also protected the emotional state." In other words, the strength of the unpleasant emotional reaction, the feelings associated with it and the thoughts about it were kept intact and unaltered when respondents went to sleep with the unsettling images fresh in their mind. In fact, some of the respondents stated that their negative emotions were amplified and even worse on second viewing.

The lesson here is that when something traumatic happens, even if it is virtual (such as fears or emotions from watching a movie), it is best to stay awake and not sleep it off. According to Spenser, "This study suggests the biological response we have after trauma might actually be healthy. Perhaps letting people go through a period of insomnia before feeding them sleeping meds is actually beneficial." It's beneficial for the short term because the body does need sleep to repair — especially after a traumatic incident. Therefore, it is best to try to find perspective and reframe the way you see the event before sleeping. "The Headache Relief Action Plan" offers many such emotional-release methods and techniques, many of which are introduced in the next chapter.

CHAPTER REVIEW

- Never underestimate the power of restful sleep as a way to reduce pain and inflammation, all while allowing your body to repair itself.
- Actively practice the "Eight Tips for a Restful Night's sleep.".
- If you have difficulty falling or staying asleep, use the "progressive relaxation" technique outlined in this chapter.
- Wrong sleeping causes pain due to nerve impingement and muscle spasm. Sleeping on your back or side with arms below your head will correct this.
- Don't sleep on negative emotions; use one of the psychosomatic release techniques outlined in this book.

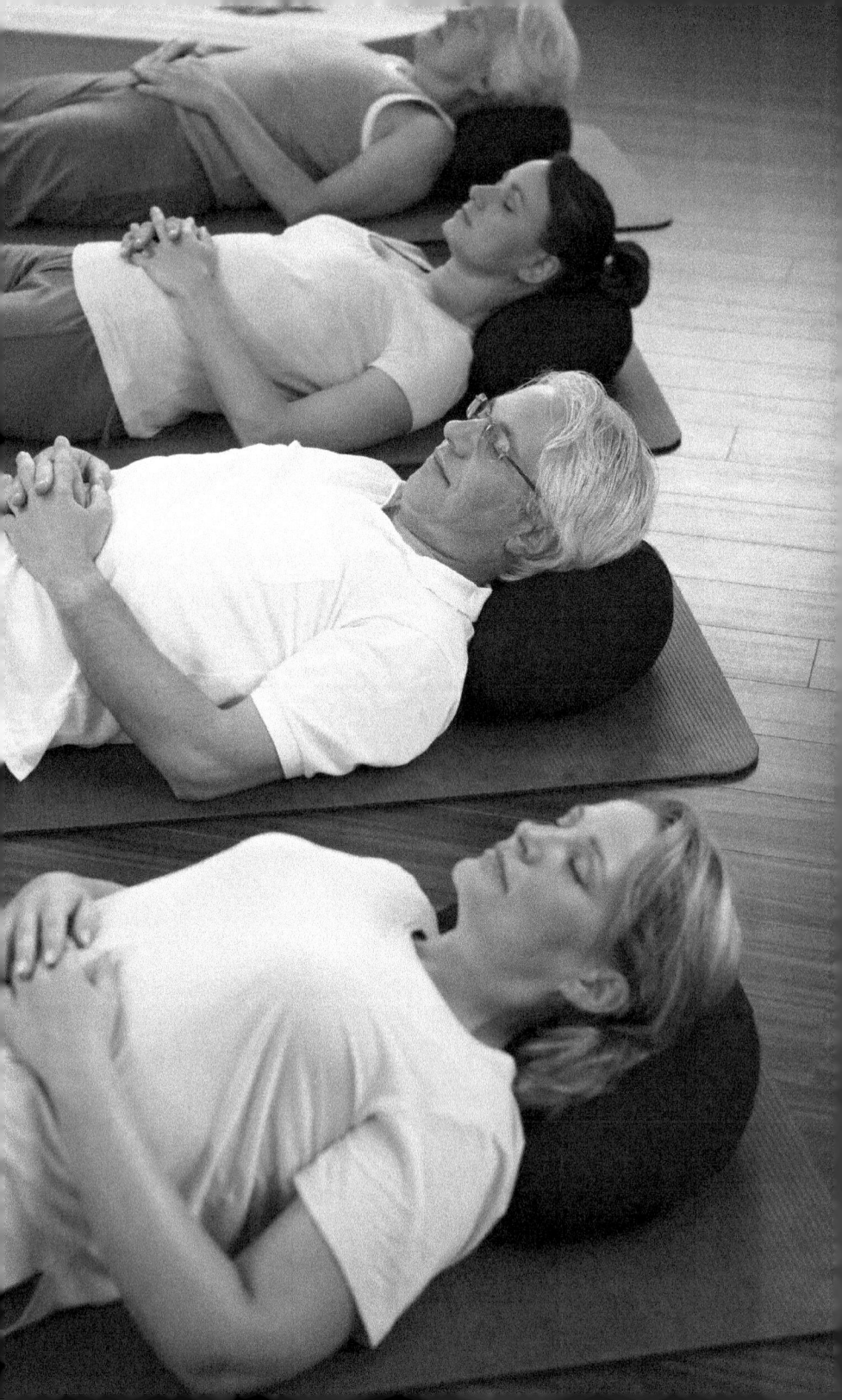

CHAPTER 14

RELEASING THE PAIN BODY FOR HEADACHE RELIEF

For some people, the cause of their acute and chronic headaches is psychosomatic; meaning, *the issue is related to both mind and body* and how they *interact*. What I am talking about is how negative thought patterns can keep you from recovering from illness, and how they also can create your headache condition or make it worse. They do this by creating a mild oxygen deprivation in the body that hampers the health of cells and muscles. This causes restriction of blood vessels and contraction of muscles. What's more, the constant worry, and stressful or upset state causes constriction of muscles and blood vessels, which trigger migraines and headaches.

You know, it's those tight shoulders you feel when your boss reprimands you or your loved one yells and you hold back negative feelings. It's the repression of such negative feelings that does the damage or at least initiates a sequence of things that later causes headaches (like overeating and weight gain, lack of exercise, stiff muscles, etc.).

If the physical body has been treated in every safe way imaginable but to no avail, perhaps looking at your thoughts and your emotions – a psychosomatic root cause – may be the next logical step for you. Below we look at several of the safest, easiest, and most powerful mind-body systems for eradicating chronic pain associated with repressed negative thoughts and emotions. This is what Eckhart Tolle calls "the pain body." I like his term, so we'll begin with his insights.

ECKHART TOLLE'S PAIN BODY

Eckhart Tolle is a modern, enlightened person and teacher of all things related to spirituality and enlightenment. According to him, the "pain-body" is the accumulation of psychological distress that is held in the physical body and comes out at various times, causing poor behavior, violence, road rage, and shows up more consistently as chronic pain. According to Tolle:

> *"The pain body that is ready to feed can use the most insignificant event as a trigger, something somebody says or does, or even a thought. If you live alone or there is nobody around at the time, the pain-body will feed on your thoughts."*[1]

Everything in the universe is an expression of energy. Energy is vibration, and we are surrounded by energy; we are made up of it. The vibratory rate of healthy humans is different than that of unhealthy humans. The trick is to raise your vibration to resonate at rates that are in the healthy human spectrum. This means adjusting how you think and what you choose to think about; as well as how you view the world, the words you use, the music you listen to, and the food you eat. Tolle explains it this way:

> *"Thoughts have their own range of frequencies, with negative thoughts at the lower end of the scale and positive thoughts at the higher. The vibrational frequency of the pain-body resonates with that of negative thoughts, which is why only those thoughts can feed the pain-body. Emotion from the pain-body quickly gains control of your thinking, and once your mind has been taken over by the painbody, your thinking becomes negative."*

Whether you "believe in" a "pain body" or not, the mechanism of the mind affecting the body is well established. And the connection between stress, anxiety, depression, anger, resentment, and other repressed emotions are known triggers of headaches and migraines. This is perhaps one of the greatest causes of chronic headaches and chronic pain in general. "The Headache Relief Action Plan" includes a number of powerful (and perhaps unusual) mind-body methods for changing energetic frequency, creating new neural pathways in the brain, and changing upsetting feelings into objective acknowledgement of the situations around which feelings form, without the accompanying pain trigger.

I have been asked often why I teach these methods for dealing with headaches associated with psychosomatic issues rather than directing people into talk therapy or counseling sessions. Well, simply put: not only does therapy take too long, it's not effective. Let's look at why.

PSYCHOTHERAPY IS NOT WORKING

There's an old joke in the movie, *Annie Hall*, where the character Alvy Singer is having a meal with Annie's family. Mom Hall says, "Ann tells us that you've been seeing a psychiatrist for fifteen years." Alvy responds, jokingly, "Yes. I'm making excellent progress. Pretty soon when I lie down on his couch, I won't have to wear the lobster bib."

That quote is one of those classic movie lines. But as it turns out, it's no joke. Talk therapy just does not work as well as they'd hoped it would back in the 70's. In 2015, researchers uncovered that—for depression at least—it is actually 25% less effective than reported.

A research team led by Ellen Driessen of VU University in Amsterdam conducted a systematic review and meta-analysis of the U.S. National Institutes of Health-funded trials conducted between 1972 and 2008.[2] The research team "assessed directly the extent of study publication bias in trials examining the efficacy of psychological treatment for depression."

They uncovered 55 funded grants that began trials, but did not publish results and then requested the data from the researchers. The results showed that talk therapies, like cognitive behavior therapy and interpersonal therapy—while effective—were indeed less effective than previously believed. "Among comparisons to control conditions, adding unpublished studies to published studies reduced the psychotherapy effect size point estimate by 25%."

So while drug therapy and talk therapy do indeed help some patients, they are less effective as previously believed and are best used in conjunction with other treatments. In the case of chronic painful conditions like headaches, mind-body techniques are a better bet.

EMOTIONAL FREEDOM TECHNIQUE (EFT)

Based on a method known as Thought Field Therapy and also on acupuncture theory, EFT relieves pain and illness by addressing the connection between your body's subtle energies, your emotions and your health.

This therapeutic method is similar to transcranial magnetic stimulation, but goes deeper in its explanation of what causes the emotional imbalances. EFT practitioners believe that disturbances in your energy field cause the negative emotions, which then cause your symptoms. Essentially, EFT teaches methods of looking in specific directions, touching and pressing your face and arms in certain places to open the energy channels and rebalance what is out of balance. This then allows your body to return to normal functioning and for your signs and symptoms to decrease or disappear.

It appears that anyone can learn and use Emotional Freedom Technique by taking a course, reading a book or going through the tutorials on EFT websites.

EYE MOVEMENT DESENSITIZATION AND REPROCESSING (EMDR)

Eye movement desensitization and reprocessing (EMDR) may not be as widely known as the Emotional Freedom Technique (EFT) discussed above, but it is another unique therapy that has received a good deal of press lately. EMDR is among the most peer-reviewed and has been researched extensively. EMDR's effectiveness has been validated in more than two dozen randomized studies. EMDR triggers an innate, natural stress release process in the brain that often produces rapid and long-lasting changes even when other types of treatment have failed. Trauma takes many forms, including auto accidents, physical abuse, psychological abuse, stress, losing a loved one, and many others. These can be repressed and trigger a psychosomatic response.

"The symptoms of trauma show up in many different ways," says Kalie Marino[3], a Pennsylvania social worker, mind-body healer and EMDR practitioner, "including personality changes, aggressive and avoidance behaviors, withdrawal, fearful reactions, re-experiencing traumas, memory and concentration problems, sleep disorders, and nervous habits."

I made an appointment to speak with Marino after reading a book titled *Getting Past Your Past.*[4] According to Marino, EMDR has been shown to be "the most effective and thoroughly researched method ever used in the treatment of trauma. EMDR triggers an innate, natural stress release process in the brain that often produces rapid and long-lasting changes even when other types of treatment have failed."

Marino tells me that despite common understanding, time does not heal all wounds. In fact, it reinforces old ones while creating new ones:

> *"Unhealed wounds are emotional buttons that get pushed involuntarily, triggering inappropriate emotional and sometimes physical reactions that adversely affect our lives and can get worse over time. By activating the natural, information-processing system of the brain, people achieve their therapeutic goals at a rapid rate with recognizable changes that don't disappear over time."*

In other words, EMDR does not help you forget the incident, but it removes the "emotional charge" associated with it. The process allows you to recall the event and tell about it as a statement of fact, without bringing up all the past emotion, turmoil, fear and other feelings once associated with it. And by releasing those emotional feelings from the negative event, its memory ceases to trigger new, negative emotions and beliefs in the present time.

EMDR is constructed in eight phases that focus on a three-part protocol. It's safe, easy, and effective. If you are struggling with past events, physically or emotionally traumatic, then give EMDR a try.

THE SEDONA METHOD

Pioneered by Lester Levenson, The Sedona Method is a powerful yet easy-to-learn technique that teaches you how to "let go" of unwanted emotions in an instant. These emotions cause ill health, pain, and suffering. In essence, The Sedona Method consists of a series of questions you ask yourself that lead your awareness to what you are feeling in the moment and gently guide you into the experience of "letting go."

This method is easy to do because there are only a few steps necessary to accomplish the release of new or decades-old, pent-up negative emotions. With so many successes, this again points to the vital role that the mind and emotions play in the pain cycle and the ill effects we suffer in our bodies – those psychosomatic illnesses.

The effectiveness of The Sedona Method has been validated by respected scientific researchers at major universities and the MONY Corporation. In fact, if you're not feeling happy, confident, and relaxed at least 90% of the time, chances are your ailments are manifestations of these less-than-great emotions.

Sedona literature puts it this way: "It is our limiting emotions that prevent us from creating and maintaining the lives that we choose. We abdicate our decision-making ability to them. We even imagine that our emotions can dictate to us who we are supposed to be. This is made apparent in our use of language. Have you ever said to someone, 'I am angry,' or, 'I am sad'? When we speak like this, we are saying to those around us and to ourselves, without realizing it, that we are our anger, or we are our grief. We relate to others and ourselves as though we are our feelings. In fact, we even invent whole stories of why we feel the way we feel in order to justify or explain this misperception of our identity."

If you've tried other mental techniques, therapy or meditation, you know it is difficult to create change. But The Sedona Method's "releasing method" operates on the "feeling" level, which makes it easy to do. It teaches you to "let go" of years of mental programs and accumulated feelings in just seconds.

TENSION MYOSITIS SYNDROME (TMS)

Tension Myositis Syndrome (TMS) is a relatively unknown and somewhat recent health diagnostic category. It was first theorized in the 1970s by John Sarno, M.D., as being a psychosomatic or mind-body disorder: a musculoskeletal neurological disorder created by the mind and emotions that changes one's physiology and causes pain and other symptoms.

Essentially, it is believed that stress and repressed emotions like anger and anxiety are the root cause of chronic pain and a host of other disorders. The theory of TMS, though not widely accepted in mainstream medicine yet, contends that repressed emotional triggers affect the nervous system which, in turn, slows blood flow to muscles, nerves and connective tissue. It basically causes a reaction or process that starves the body of oxygen, causing pain. This pain then becomes the location of focus and concern, alleviating the need (superficially) for dealing with the stress, anxiety, and other emotional issues at hand. TMS case studies show that as the emotional components are dealt with successfully, the physical ailments that were before intractable, disappear almost instantly.

While pain in general (low back pain in particular) seems to be the most common symptom of TMS, it is not the only one. Generalized stiffness and numbness and tingling in the body or limbs are also associated with the syndrome. Flare-ups from painful to severe come and go at different times, showing the correlation of symptoms to (perhaps) the emotional upset state of the individual at any given time.

Many who experience the problems of chronic pain, tension headache, fibromyalgia, irritable bowel syndrome (IBS), constipation, arm pain, temporal mandibular joint dysfunction (TMJD), and tinnitus (ringing in the ears) have had difficulty finding relief or cure from mainstream approaches. They may have the basis or root of their symptoms in TMS.

Here are four short passages from Sarno's book *Healing Back Pain*[5] that are interesting, informative, and thought-provoking:

- "TMS is equivalent to peptic ulcer, spastic colitis, constipation, tension headache, migraine headache, cardiac palpitations, eczema, allergic rhinitis (hay fever), prostatitis (often), ringing in the ears (often), and dizziness (often)."

- "I believe these disorders are interchangeable and equivalent of each other because many of them are found to occur historically in patients with TMS, sometimes at the same time, but often in tandem."

- "Equivalence is also suggested by the fact that patients often report resolution of one of these disorders when the TMS pain goes away. This happens most commonly with hay fever. I teach patients that all the conditions on the list serve the same purpose psychologically."

- "Experience with TMS, and these related conditions, suggests that there may be a common denominator, anxiety perhaps, that can bring on any of these disorders. In that case, some other emotion, anger for example, may be the primary one that may in turn induce anxiety, which then brings on the symptom."

The first step in treating TMS requires patient education. Physicians generally provide audio and written materials or recommend lectures. Education teaches the patient various aspects of the condition and reassures them that physical symptoms do not occur because of typical disease processes, physical injury or re-injury.

Another treatment modality physicians may use for treating TMS involves keeping a daily journal and writing about circumstances that might have created repressed emotional stress. After identifying a list of possible contributing factors, TMS physicians require that patients write an essay for each problem area. Longer essays allow patients to explore the issue in greater detail.

Part of TMS treatment also requires that patients live as if symptom-free. This is putting the proverbial cart before the horse, but is an effective way of "thinking from the end" and envisioning yourself in the headache-free state you seek to achieve. It's using the mind to affect the body in a positive way.

HYPNOSIS

Nothing is more powerful than teaching your brain how to control pain and encourage healing. There are many forms of hypnosis and in some states only licensed psychologists can perform hypnosis on patients. The basic idea of hypnosis is to switch off the ideas in the mind that prevent one from achieving their goals. And thoughts like, "I am always in pain" and "Nothing ever helps" are negative mantras that keep one's mind and body

Releasing the Pain Body for Headache Relief

locked in the pain cycle. The sooner these thoughts are released and replaced with positive ones, the faster the pain relief and recovery begin.

Look online and see what is available in your area, but be sure that "pain" is on the top of their list of specialties rather than hidden under a dozen other areas like smoking, anxiety, weight loss, and others. Good hypnosis audio programs from reputable companies like The Hypnosis Network can also help you.

BAUD THERAPY DEVISE

The BAUD, or Bio Acoustical Utilization Device, is a new and powerful therapy tool. Invented by Dr. Frank Lawlis, a pioneer in the field of medical psychology, the BAUD is an FDA-cleared and registered device based on the latest discoveries of neuroscience. The BAUD's technology utilizes specially designed sound frequencies and waveforms to quickly stimulate neural plasticity in a highly-targeted way.

The BAUD is a neuromodulation device that works through neuroacoustic stimulation. It is unique because it doesn't require an external monitor. The client's sensations are used to monitor their neural response, and the client tunes the frequencies to achieve a desired result. In essence, the client's brain becomes the monitor. This provides a much more targeted and effective result and clients often see dramatic results in as little as one 20-minute session.

While the BAUD's exact mechanism of action is still being researched, it seems to rapidly stimulate a parasympathetic response in very specific brain areas associated with the target problem based on results so far. This brings neural function out of an aroused level or sympathetic state, and produces often dramatic relief of the problem symptoms.

As therapists know, changing some negative feelings or compulsions is extremely difficult since the source is often unconscious. The brain areas negatively stimulated over many years can become stuck in a sympathetic, aroused response state. This energy then drives all sorts of unwanted urges or feelings or even physical symptoms. The client's attempts to change are difficult because they are fighting their own neural "programming."

The BAUD is effective in three main categories of problems: emotional issues, urges or impulses, and physical symptoms like pain. This covers a wide variety of individual problems and we are continually discovering new applications for the BAUD.

We know from brain scans that merely shifting mental attention from one thing to another will "light up" different parts of the brain as neural activity increases. It is these active areas that the BAUD affects most strongly, creating a response that regulates, or normalizes the neural activity.

This means that any problem the client can focus on is potentially one the BAUD can improve. The BAUD provides relief in a way that most clients have never experienced. It gives them a powerful, pinpointed way to address the inner, neural source of their outer problem. They can focus on general anxiety or target any specific fear that limits them: heights, confined spaces, intimacy or even simply asking for a raise. They can reduce their appetite in general or eliminate only carb cravings.

And it doesn't take long to see results. A typical BAUD session may last from 15 to 20 minutes. Immediately after a session, many clients report feeling a profound improvement in issues that have plagued them for years, even a lifetime. While individual results vary, the relief they experience from just one session tends to be enduring, and the negative feelings diminish more with each subsequent session.

CHAPTER REVIEW

- Some people's acute and chronic pain is not related to a traumatic injury or headache; rather it is psychosomatic, meaning it is related to the way the mind and body interact.
- Pent up, repressed anger and emotions "lock" pain into the body.
- If the physical body has been treated in every safe way imaginable but without improvement, looking at your thoughts and emotions – a psychosomatic cause – may be the next logical step toward relief from pain.
- Psychotherapy has been proven to not work as quickly or effectively as we were led to believe.
- Thankfully, we have many safe, easy, and powerful mind/body methods for eradicating chronic pain associated with negative thoughts and emotions.
- I recommend The Sedona Method, EFT, EMDR, Tension Myositis Syndrome (TMS), hypnosis, and BAUD Therapy.

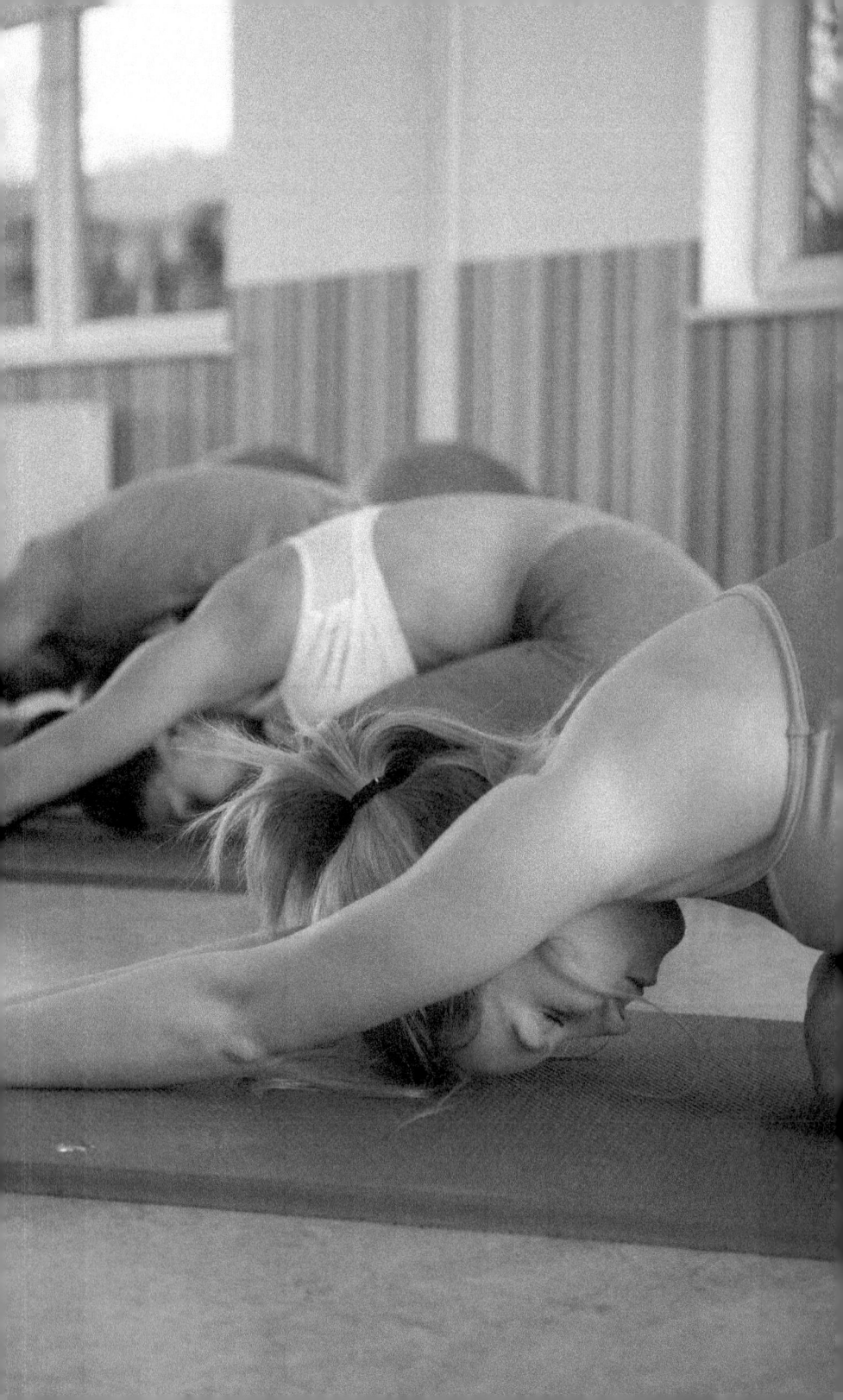

CHAPTER 15

STRETCHING AND BODYWORK FOR HEADACHE RELIEF

We know that tension-type headaches are caused by muscle contractions and pinched nerves, which not only decrease blood flow and oxygen flow in the body, but also cause structural misalignment and nerve ending irritation.

A sore neck and tense shoulders are common among those who spend hours a day seated at a desk or behind the wheel of a vehicle and in those who, regardless of vocation, harbor stress and anxiety in their body. This causes not only nerve pain but muscle contractions in the base of the skull which can cause severe head pain that then can trigger a migraine headache. It is therefore important that we keep the body relaxed and supple through a program of general stretching with specific focus given to the neck, shoulders, spine and hips. These are the areas most affected by poor posture and unreleased stresses and tensions, thus triggering muscle-contraction or tension-type headaches in those who are susceptible to them.

In this chapter, we'll look at correcting somatic imbalances; that is, postural changes in the upper back, shoulder and neck, that cause spasm, inflammation, nerve impingement, reduction in blood flow, and pain. In other words, the stresses on the body through poor posture and our psychological states, which cause a chain of events that trigger headaches and migraine. If not balanced, these become part of our life and chronic headaches are a result. In the sections that follow, we'll look at what these imbalances are, how to correct them ourselves with area-specific stretches, and, lastly, how to gain more global relaxation and release through various practitioner-based bodywork therapies.

Many who suffer chronic headaches find it difficult to exercise because they are either in too much pain or have limited range of motion. In such cases, attending a series of hands-on bodywork sessions can really help loosen the body, align the system, free the nerves, and awaken the energy. Stretching and bodywork therapies do wonders for these headache triggers.

Let's first look at area-specific stretching you can easily do on your own at any time you feel tense, to release tension and impingement resulting from mental and emotional stress, and correct the every-present forward head posture. This has become a common disorder since cell phone and iPads were in wide use. The stretching series presented here offer fast relief in the moment. We'll also review several of the best bodywork therapies for headaches and migraines.

CORRECTING FORWARD HEAD POSTURE (FHP)

Forward head posture (FHP) is one of the most common postural problems we experience on a chronic basis and a direct trigger for headaches. Today it is commonly called "text neck" by practitioners, because of the vast increase in treatments for the conditions since the popularity of looking down at iPads and cell phones all day, texting, and gaming. It is our modern lifestyle that's responsible for it—as we'll see in a minute. In essence, FHP is the result of either repetitive forward head movement or the carrying (holding) of the head in a position that is forward of the shoulder plum-line.

Forward head posture can be caused by many things. Here is a list of the five more common ones:

1) Looking down toward your hands while typing or reading
2) Looking down while playing games or texting on the phone or iPad
3) Sitting improperly with shoulders rounded and back hunched
4) Driving with your head more than 2 to 3 inches from the headrest
5) Carrying a backpack or heavy purse slung over one shoulder

These are not all the causes of FHP, but enough to make the point. The problem is that repeated forward and/or downward facing postures cause concurrent hypotonic (lengthening) and hypertonic (shortening) of several major muscles (i.e., lavater, rhomboid, trapezious, pectoral), degeneration of cervical (neck) vertebrae, and irritation of the cervical nerves.

Did you know that pinched or irritated nerves, tightened muscles, and isometric contraction all cause pain as a result of the stagnation of blood, fluids, and energy? As you recall from Chapter 7, where there is blockage or stagnation, there is pain.

SIMPLE STRETCHING SERIES

Now that we've identified a single, underlying cause of many problems, the next step is correcting the problem. And what better way to do this than following the simple idea of returning the body to homeostasis. That is, rebalancing what is imbalanced. Here are four simple things you can do to correct (balance) Forward Head posture.

For the purposes of headache prevention, it is not necessary to achieve the great flexibility required of some sports. Rather, it is important only to *relax*, become supple, and achieve a general sense of "feeling good." Therefore, do not strain or worry while stretching, just relax and let the stretch happen *of its own accord*. It is best, then, to engage in progressive relaxation with full range of muscle-joint motion.

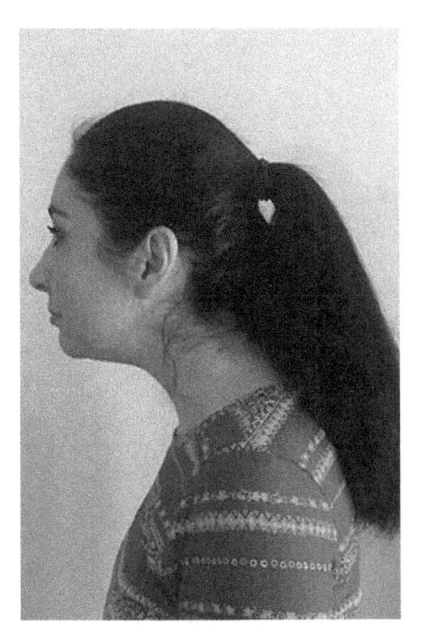

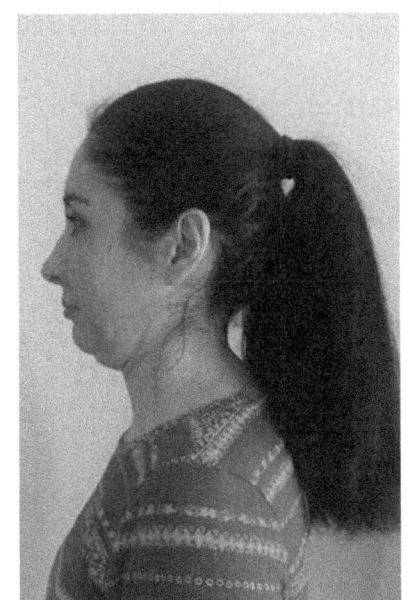

Figure 1   Figure 2

Chin Tuck

Stand or sit upright and hold your shoulders straight. Stick your chin out to the front, hold for three seconds (fig. 1). Pull your chin in as far back as it will go, hold for three seconds (fig. 2). Repeat six times. Do this three times per day.

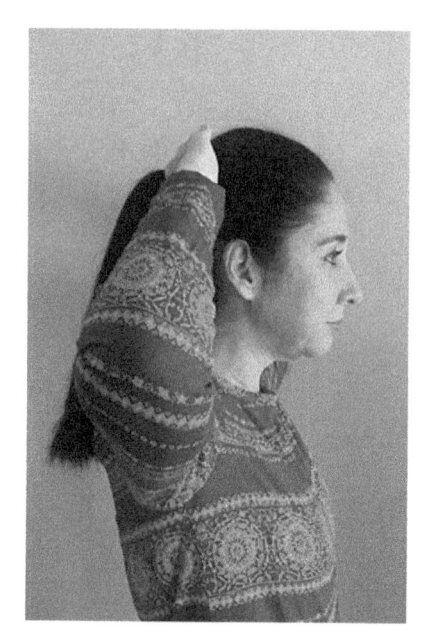

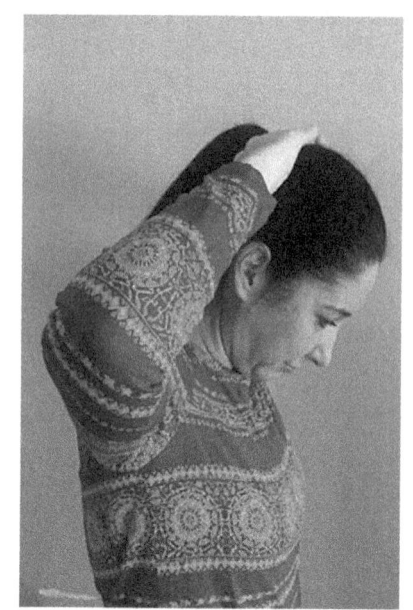

Figure 1   *Figure 2*

Chin to Chest Stretch

Stand or sit upright and overlap your fingers and place both hands behind your head (fig. 1). Use your hands to push your head down so your chin goes toward your chest (fig. 2). Do NOT lower your head and then press with your hands, as this defeats the idea of the stretch. Hold the stretch for 20 seconds and return to the upright position. You should feel a stretch between your shoulders. Repeat three times. Do this three times per day.

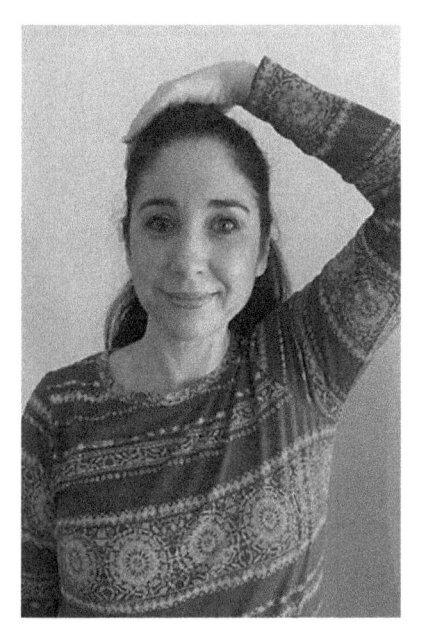

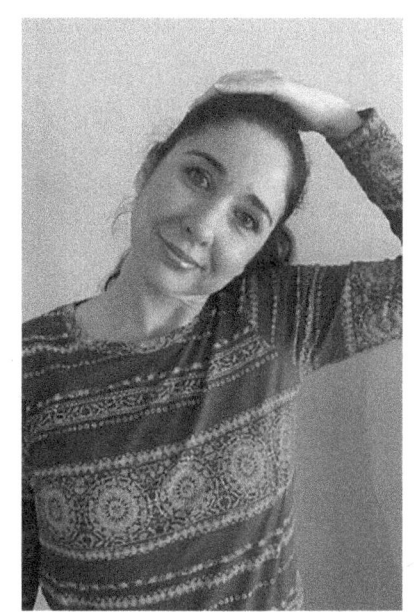

Figure 1 *Figure 2*

Ear to Shoulder

Stand or sit erect with shoulders level. Reach your right hand over your head and place your fingers on your left temple (Fig. 1). Gently pull your head to the side, keeping your head straight and not twisted. You want to pull your right ear down toward your right shoulder (fig. 2). Hold the stretch for 20 seconds and return to the upright position. You should feel a stretch along the left side of your neck. Repeat three times and then repeat three times on the other side. Do this three times per day.

Figure 1 *Figure 2*

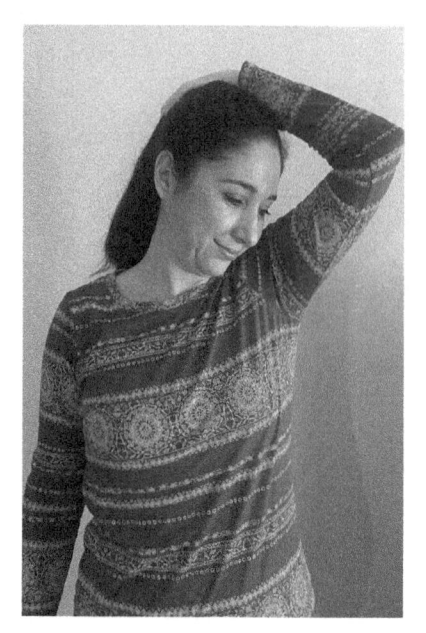

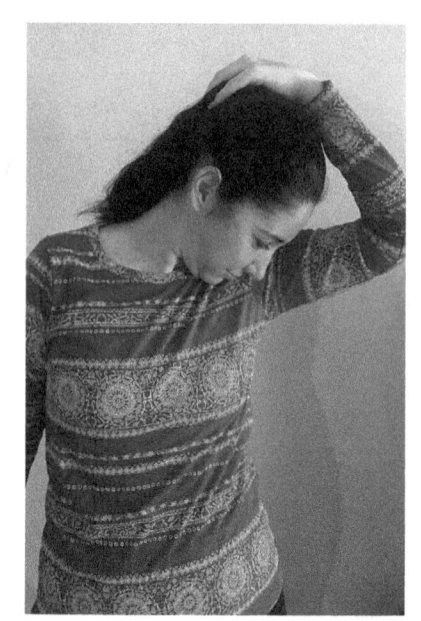

Nose-to-Underarm Stretch

From a standing or seated position, turn your head to the right, reach your right hand over the top of your head, holding the back of it (fig. 1). Slowly pull your head diagonally down, as if trying to pull your nose into your underarm (fig. 2). Hold the stretch for a count of three. Next, slowly push your head back against your hand, slowly returning it to the starting position. Repeat on the other side. Now repeat this sequence 3 more times.

Stretching and Bodywork for Headache Relief

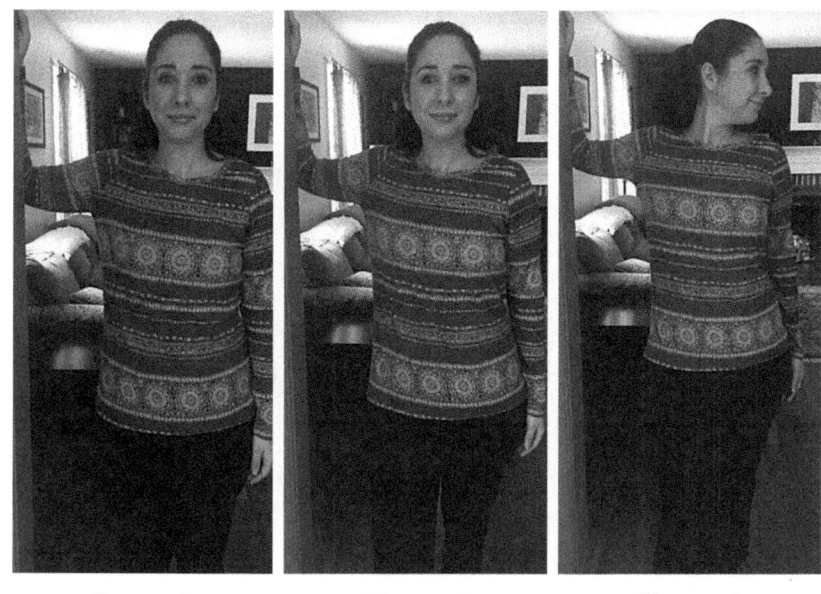

Figure 1   Figure 2   Figure 3

Doorway Stretch

Stand with both feet parallel behind (but in the center of) a door frame. Place one arm 90-degrees along the side of the doorframe facing you (fig. 1). If your right arm is touching the frame, then your right foot takes a long step forward. (fig. 2) Be sure to bend your knee, as if you were really trying to walk forward. You should feel a nice stretch across your chest. If not, turn your body to the left more (fig. 3). Hold for 20 seconds. Repeat three times and then switch sides. Do this three times per day.

Here are a few simple ways to adjust your daily activities to prevent FHP from taking hold in your body—or returning after balance is achieved:

- ✓ Make sure the top of your computer screen is level with your eyes, and about two feet away from your face.
- ✓ Be sure to carry a backpack squarely over both shoulders to balance the weight distribution.
- ✓ If you carry a heavy purse or duffel bag, it's better to sling it diagonally across the torso.
- ✓ Have ample lower back support while sitting or lying for prolonged periods, as a lax position leads to slouching, which can lead to FHP.

MASSAGE THERAPY

If done correctly, massage therapy can work wonders for people in pain. It may not always be the best choice, and may not work for everyone, but most people will get great results if the massage therapist has a good understanding of the human body, muscle imbalances, and how to work with them.

Massage improves circulation, and this is a big component of pain relief. A clear fluid called lymph circulates around our body's tissues. At the same time, you may have inflammation, which is an immune response to injury or infection that causes pain, redness, heat, and swelling in the affected area. When lymph and inflammation start to accumulate in the body, the excess fluid puts pressure on blood vessels and circulation decreases, limiting blood flow. As the pressure increases, it irritates the nerves, which cause pain. By helping the body remove excess lymph and inflammation, massage therapy can assist with blood flow, which will reduce the pressure that is irritating the nerves and get rid of your pain.

Massage also provides a number of other benefits, including relaxing the muscles, improving your range of motion, decreasing mental and emotional stress, improving your sleep, and increasing your production of endorphins (which will improve your mood). Is it any wonder you feel like a million bucks after a massage?

There are literally hundreds of styles of massage. Which one is best for you will depend on your comfort levels. Standard massage is good because it moves toxins through the body and is relaxing. But it often does not correct structural problems or offer enough correction in the range of motion. Remember, it is limited range of motion and inflammation that cause pain.

TRIGGER POINT THERAPY

Trigger points are small contraction knots that develop in muscle and tissue when an area of the body is stressed, "frozen," injured or overworked. Sitting for too long or even restricting your movements because of pain or the type of work you do, can cause tiny landmines about the size of a dime to erupt deep in your muscle tissue. These are called trigger points, and they can occur in your back, arms, legs, and feet.

Massage therapy is usually not as effective once trigger points have a hold on your body and are the cause of your pain. What is needed for relief here is sufficient, deep sustained pressure to the "knotted-up area." As the trigger point is worked out, your body will undergo soft tissue release, allowing for increased blood flow, a reduction in muscle spasm, and the break-up of scar tissue. It will also help remove any build-up of toxic, metabolic waste.

The good news is, with deep and focused pressure to these areas you can release this pain from your body. What is needed is sufficient, deep sustained pressure to the "knotted-up area." As the trigger point is compressed, your body will undergo soft tissue release, allowing for increased blood flow, a reduction in muscle spasm, and the break-up of scar tissue. It also helps remove any build-up of toxic metabolic waste.

Trigger point therapy can be received at the hands of a manual therapist trained in its method. There are also good self-treatment trigger point systems that can work just as well or better. With a self-treatment trigger point system, you can apply pressure to the trigger points every day or several times per day until relief is found.

With trigger point therapy, your body also undergoes a neurological release, reducing the pain signals to the brain and resetting your neuromuscular system to restore its proper function. In other words, everything will again work the way it should.

The basic idea is simply to apply sustained pressure on the trigger point area for a set period of time on a regular basis, usually about 90 seconds per point. If you cannot locate a "trigger point specialist" among the body workers in your area, trying looking for "acupressure" as it is another name for it.

THAI YOGA MASSAGE

Thai yoga massage (TYM) is a gentle method of hands-on bodywork that is based on rhythmic and measured compression and release of the muscles. It successfully combines assisted stretching and yoga postures from either a seated or lying position. In general, massage different oils are rubbed on naked body. But because of the nature of the Thai-yoga techniques, the body is fully clothed in loose fitting garments and no oils are used.

The TYM therapist holds different body parts to gently stretch them, press them or compress them in a slow and rhythmic fashion that releases tension and fosters relaxation. Sometimes, the practitioner (who is usually a petite woman), will hold onto rails and use her feet and body weight to massage the back. The massage follows a sequence from head to toe and releases the energy lines and connective tissue to induce a deep level of somatic correction, relaxation, and to free up the body's range of motion.

For those in pain with stiff muscles and joints and with limited range of motion, Thai-yoga massage is a blessing. Unfortunately, its practitioners are few and far between, so be sure to check local massage therapy locations and the Internet.

TUI-NA THERAPY

China's 3,000 year tradition of bodywork known as Tui-Na is based on acupuncture theory. It is a rigorous therapy that loosens muscles and joints, relaxes tendons, reduces swelling and relieves pain by promoting the circulation of energy, blood, and lymph. It combines techniques of manually pushing, pulling, grasping, pressing, and manipulating the muscles, tendons and bones to work through stiffness or injury.

In the Tui-Na technique, pressure is applied to the meridians (energy lines) and specific points on them (acu-points) that affects the flow of Qi (vital energy), and helps it move freely and evenly throughout the body. When your body is balanced, you feel relaxed and full of energy. You are free from stiffness, aches or pain.

A word of caution, Tui-Na is not for the timid or those in acute pain. It should not be confused with a nice, relaxing massage. It is vigorous and sometimes painful… but then, it is a therapy based on correcting a problem.

CHOOSING THE BEST METHOD

The above-mentioned alternative therapies are just a handful of those which are able to bring relief from pain and illness by correcting energetic imbalances in the body. They are based on thousands of years of trial-and-error application and have an amazing track record of success.

If you have tried just about everything and are still in pain, then you might want to ditch the mainstream idea of health. Instead, open your mind to these traditional ideas of the body being composed of energy, and that energy vibrating at various frequencies, positively and negatively affecting the mind, body, spirit and organs.

Pain is caused when there is a blockage of this energy. These practices unblock your inherent life energies. Give them a try… pain relief may be just around the corner.

CHAPTER REVIEW

- Self-stretching on the neck and shoulders is a great way to reduce stress and tension that impinge nerves and slow blood flow, causing headaches. When you feel stressed or tense in the neck or shoulders, follow the stretching sequence presented herein.

- Bodywork therapies utilize the hands of a practitioner on your body to effect change in a positive way

- Because of weakness, pain, or lost range of motion, many people don't feel able to exercise, and need a little help moving forward

- Attending a series of bodywork sessions helps to loosen the body, align the system, free the nerves and awaken the energy - giving you relief.

- Of all bodywork therapies, I recommend self-stretching, massage, trigger point, Thai-yoga massage, and Tui Na therapies

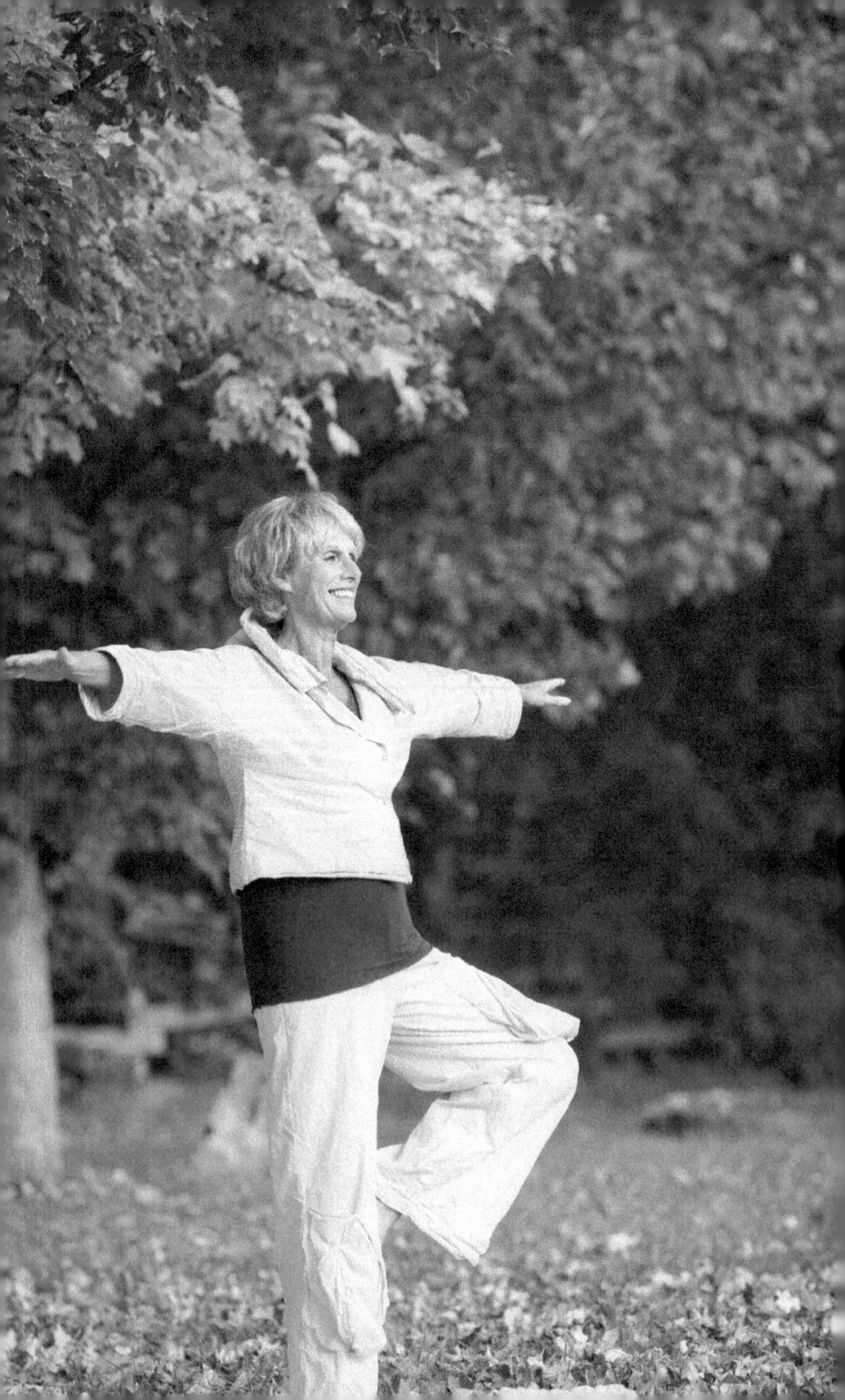

CHAPTER 16

ANCIENT EXERCISES FOR HEADACHE RELIEF

Engaging in the right type and level of exercise for at least 20 minutes at a time for several days per week is a powerful tool in preventing headaches. In one activity, we are able to increase blood flow, decrease blood sugars and fats, burn calories, reduce adipose tissue, increase oxygen flow to the brain, increase our resting metabolism, loosen the musculoskeletal system, and detoxify the body while improving digestion and eliminative functions. Without a doubt, exercise is an essential part of the integrated mind-body approach to headache prevention.

THE HEALING POWER OF EXERCISE

The utilization of stored energy is what propels the human body and gives it the fuel necessary to do such basic things as stand, bend, and lift objects. This energy we derive mainly from the complex carbohydrates we eat, which are stored in the body as sugars and fats.

Energy is released in the body through the process of respiration. During any physical activity, we breathe in air.

Oxygen from that breath moves into the bloodstream where it is transported to the organs and utilized to burn the stored sugar and fat "fuel." The waste product of this process is carbon dioxide, and this passes back into the bloodstream, back into the lungs and then is removed from the body on exhale. The greater the duration and higher the intensity of physical exercise, the greater the amount of oxygen is taken into the body and moved into the bloodstream, and the more carbon dioxide waste is expelled from the body.

There are basically two types of exercise, or methods of utilizing stored sugars and fat: anaerobic and aerobic. Anaerobic exercise does not require oxygen, instead it burns glucose (derived from carbohydrates) from the muscle's store of sugar reserves (glycogen). However, these reserves are quickly depleted and the body must then draw its energy from stored body fat and blood fat. But this action requires oxygen to work, and this type of exercise is called aerobic. Since aerobic exercise utilizes oxygen, stored glucose and fat, it is able to burn fat calories, decrease the resting heart rate, increase oxygen flow to the brain, and ease stress and muscle tension by releasing beta-endorphins, the body's natural pain reliever. Thus, both anaerobic and aerobic exercises contribute greatly to our headache prevention program.

Our aim in preventing headaches is to return the body to its natural balanced state of homeostasis. Both anaerobic exercise and aerobic exercises contribute to this by increasing both blood flow and oxygen flow which help stabilize blood vessels (by supplying a steady supply of oxygen to the brain) and normalize blood sugars and blood fats (by utilizing them for energy). And we know that dilating and constricting blood vessels and high levels of fats and sugars in the bloodstream and adipose (fat) tissue are direct causes of headaches.

Regular exercise is also a powerful tool in our efforts toward detoxification. Since prolonged physical activity activates the sweat glands, it enables elimination of wastes and toxins through the skin. Since it utilizes fats and sugars for energy it burns calories and eliminates toxins from our system. Toxins are also released through the breath and bowel functions, and both are improved through exercise.

EXERCISES AS EFFECTIVE AS DRUGS

In a three-month study, researchers at the University of Gothenburg in Sweden divided a group of over 90 women who regularly experience migraines into three subgroups: 1) One who exercised for 40 minutes three times weekly; 2) one who practiced relaxation techniques; and, 3) a third who took the drug topiramate (Topamax).

The researchers found that all three groups experienced significantly reduced migraines, suggesting that exercise and relaxation may be as effective at alleviating headaches as pharmaceuticals, but without potential side effects.

"Our conclusion is that exercise can act as an alternative to relaxations and topiramate when it comes to preventing migraines, and is particularly appropriate for patients who are unwilling or unable to take preventative medicines," said lead author Emma Varkey.

ANCIENT EXERCISES ARE HEADACHE SUFFERERS' BEST CHOICE

The key to introducing exercise into your chronic headache lifestyle is being able to engage in a set of physical movements that invigorates the body but does not trigger more pain. In my own 30+ year's battle with chronic headaches, I have learned to rely on a few ancient exercises to keep me balanced and do wonders in preventing these monsters. When considering exercises for headaches and migraine, these exercises must provide the following:

- ✓ **Promote Circulation**
- ✓ **Relax Contracted (Tight) Muscles**
- ✓ **Tone Weak Muscles**
- ✓ **Increase Range of Motion**
- ✓ **Invigorate the blood**
- ✓ **Support the Nervous System**
- ✓ **Promote Detoxification**
- ✓ **Not Make Headaches Worse**

There is also the mental and emotional component to consider, as well. Engaging in an exercise program that is or seems daunting may be overwhelming and cause you to quit too soon or not begin at all. Any health approach should incorporate an integrated mind-body theme. This is an essential component of the physical activity you choose as exercise. In addition to burning calories, increasing oxygen intake, stabilizing blood fats and sugars, and releasing feel-good hormones, you will also develop a mind-body center that helps focus your thoughts, emotions and spirit. The aftereffect of exercise is a reduction in the stress and anxiety that often accompany and trigger headaches and migraines.

I'd like to share four exercise methods that are aligned with the components mentioned above, and are enjoyable and easy to do. They will get you toned, and help you lose weight while also connecting your mind and body. These are Mindful Walking, Qigong Standing Pole, Tai Chi and Yoga.

MINDFUL WALKING

If done correctly, brisk walking can be one of the safest and most beneficial and enjoyable of exercises. Walking is an aerobic activity, but since it is low-impact there is little wear-and-tear on the joints and little (if any) triggering of headaches from the jarring action of the body experienced in high-impact aerobic exercises or jogging. Although it is a simple activity, walking actually utilizes most of the muscles of the body to propel you forward and keep you on balance while increasing respiration, heart and lung function, blood and oxygen flow, and the "burning off" of blood sugars and fats and removal of toxins and other wastes through sweat and improved eliminative functions. All of this, of course, causes a vast decrease in pain.

Walking is so simple and *ordinary*, yet in one 20-minute session you can raise HDL (good cholesterol levels), increase respiration within safe limits, sweat out toxins, release the endorphin "feel-good" hormones, improve heart function, begin reducing weight, reduce stress, promote relaxation, and improve overall endurance and body tone. Amazing!

Many of the triggers that attack your health and cause pain can be reduced or eliminated simply by walking. And this activity only requires time, as no special place needs be made to do it — although it is preferable to walk in a park as opposed to a busy city sidewalk.

Though walking in and of itself is a common activity, few of us do it properly. You must look to walking as a mind-body activity, wherein your mind is clear, emotions calm, respiration steady, and body properly aligned and relaxed with each walking step even and balanced. If you are able to integrate each of these components while walking for at least 20 minutes a day, then your walks can be considered a microcosm of an integrated mind-body approach to health and wellness ... and you will begin to derail the chronic pain cycle on your first outing.

QIGONG STANDING POLE EXERCISES

Qigong is an ancient Chinese mind-body discipline that seeks to establish a healthy body. Although such practices can appear "fluffy and soft," they are not. I have personally been studying various forms of Qigong in the United States and Asia for 30 years. I have found that while there are hundreds of Qigong practices, they all focus on the three treasures and three regulations. For the headache sufferer—especially those with chronic musculoskeletal headache triggers—the simpler the system, the better.

Qigong energy work is now quite popular in the West. Yet for centuries it has been a part of the Eastern way of life. In China, people can be found in droves in the local parks at the break of dawn practicing Qigong and Tai Chi to maintain or regain their health. Qigong are systems of concurrently exercising the body and the internal organs to stretch the body, open the meridians (energy lines), release tension, clear the mind, balance respiration, and improve the circulation of energy, blood and body fluids. All of this is achieved in relatively brief exercise sets that are simple and effective against pain, stiffness and disease.

Regular practice of Qigong exercises aid in regulating the functions of the central nervous system. Along with exercising and controlling one's mind and body, Qigong influences one's physical states and pathological conditions. While there are literally hundreds of different Qigong practices, they all have a similar theme and purpose. I will describe the method known as *zhan zhuang*, or simply the "standing pole" method. It requires only enough space to stand still, and it is so simple you will not be distracted by having to remember specific sequences of movement.

This practice is easy. Stand with your legs shoulder-width apart, and knees bent only one to two-inches with both arms bent and held at the same level. Below are three standing postures for you to do in sequence.

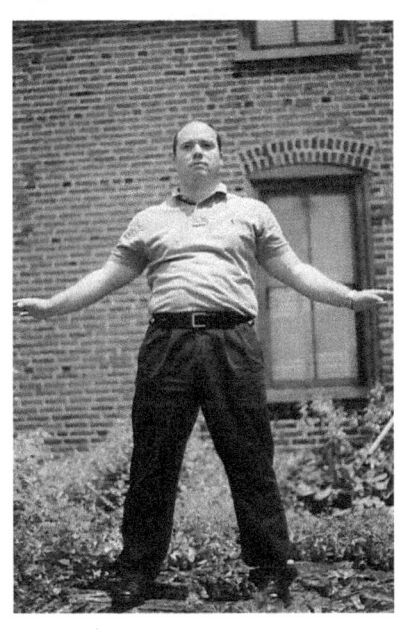

1 – Hand Floating on Water. Hold your arms out to their sides, palms facing down. Visualize that your palms are floating on water. Be sure to keep them in place and not move them during the exercise.

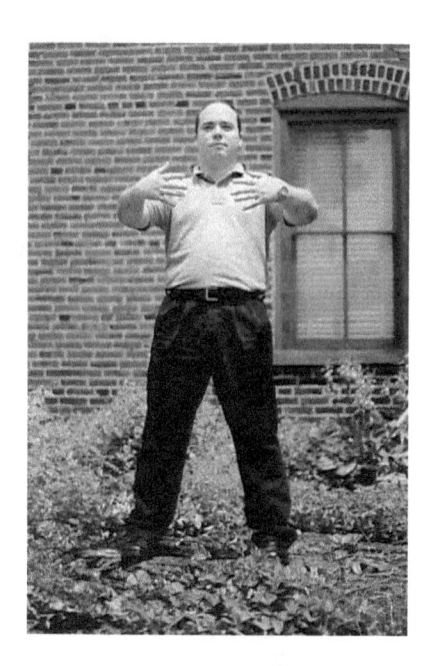

2 – Hugging a Tree. From the previous posture, slowly raise your arms to chest level while pulling them slightly inward. You want to feel as if you are hugging a tree, which is a mental image to keep your arms from coming too close to the body. Relax your hands, elbows and wrists, again like they are floating on water.

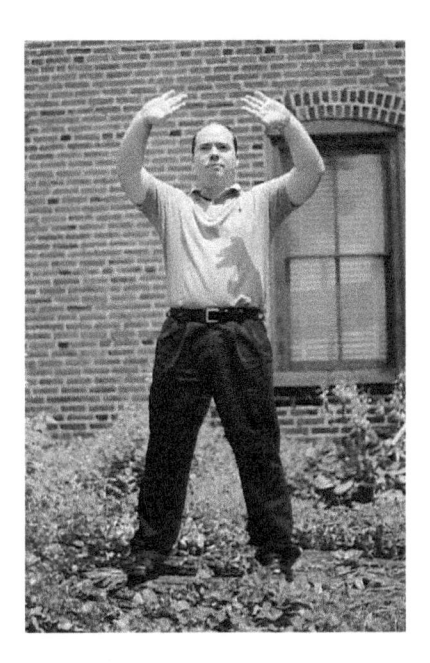

3 – Holding Up the Sky. From the previous posture, slowly rotate your palms outward while lifting your arms upward. The final position should find your hands at about forehead height, extended slightly forward and upward, as if holding up the sky from falling.

Once the posture is assumed, do the following three steps:

1. **Quiet Your Mind** by not stressing over distracting thoughts that may come – simply allow them to go freely without passing judgment.

2. **Regulate Your Respiration** by quietly breathing in and out at a steady relaxed pace. Continue doing this and enjoy yourself for the next nine minutes.

3. **Transition** to the next posture. After nine minutes, slowly move your arm position to the next posture. Do not excite your mind or move your legs, as this will distract your energy and intention.

Headaches Relieved

This sounds so simple yet there is quite a bit going on as explained in a quote from *Traditional Chinese Therapeutic Exercises – Standing Pole* by Wang Xuanjei and J.P.C. Moffett:

> "Standing pole is an exercise of the whole body. As the outer form of the body is not moved, all the internal organs settle, while all metabolic functions increase. This develops movement within non-movement, that is, unhindered internal activity and movement within external stillness. It is a non-violent and non-overburdening exercise, simultaneously providing rest and exercise, easily adaptable to any condition and encouraging development of the body's innate strengths and abilities in a natural way."[1]

You see, although it appears as if you are doing nothing, the body is really engaged in a process of physical activity. While quieting the mind and regulating respiration you are reducing stress, relaxing the cerebral cortex and rejuvenating the central nervous system. You are also working muscles by virtue of maintaining an isometric posture wherein the knees and elbows are bent, the arms are raised and this must be held steady without release until the end of the session. This elevates the heart rate without overtaxing the heart, improves the circulation of blood and oxygen throughout the body, and increases metabolic functions while releasing toxins and tension from the body.

QiGong standing pole postures are a great way to begin exercising the body and connecting your body with your mind. In times when you are in too much pain to exercise or even walk, the standing pole exercises will help rehabilitate you, help you start feeling better, and be a jumping-off point for next-level exercises. At this time, with your specific level of pain tolerance, if you can only do the standing exercises, that is ok. They have been healing people in China for centuries.

TAI CHI

Tai Chi is an ancient practice of energy cultivation and body development steeped in traditions of Chinese meditation, breathing exercises, and martial arts. Tai Chi is actually a link between QiGong breath-work exercises and Kung-fu body training. It is a mind-body discipline that strengthens mind and body while cultivating life force energy. It keeps muscles toned, tendons relaxed, joints supple, and the blood freely circulating. All of this engenders relaxation, stress relief, and pain reduction.

There are eight reasons everyone suffering from headaches and migraines should practice Tai Chi:

1. It helps clear and quiet the mind, reducing stress and anxiety while promoting focus and concentration.
2. It helps regulate the lungs and heart without taxing them, improving wellness and detoxification.
3. It helps burn calories without taxing the joints or stressing the heart, improving fitness levels while aiding in slow and steady weight loss.
4. It helps restore proper range of motion in the wrists, elbows, shoulders, hips, knees and ankles, preventing muscle spasms and neuralgic pain.
5. It helps keep the body active at a sustained rate for a period, moving blood, improving lymph drainage, moving fluids throughout the body and being a source of invigoration.

Tai Chi also has what are known as "long forms" and "short forms," referring to the number of movements in their sequence. The short form is fine for many people and is easier to learn. However, for those wanting the best of what Tai Chi offers, the long form contains more movements, takes longer and is more interesting overall. I like to think of this art as a "life study" as it combines intellectual activity (learning, remembering and perfecting the sequence), physical activity (the movements and postures themselves), moving meditation (clearing the mind and aligning the body while in motion), and QiGong energy work (combining and coordinating mind, breath and posture in motion).

Because you are holding postures with bent arms and bent knees, Tai Chi is an isometric exercise. However, because you are also moving between postures and connecting them, Tai Chi is also an isotonic exercise.

New studies conducted by Katherine Kerr, a Tai Chi teacher at Harvard Medical School, have found that Tai Chi may also help reduce or prevent disorders of memory and brain function.[2] According to Kerr:

> *"Brain plasticity arising from repeated training may be relevant, since we know that brain connections are 'sculpted' by daily experience and practice... Tai Chi is a very interesting form of training because it combines a low-intensity aerobic exercise with a complex, learned, motor sequence. Meditation, motor learning and focus have all been shown in numerous studies to be associated with training-related changes – including, in some cases, changes in actual brain structure – in specific cortical regions."*

HATHA YOGA

Yoga is an ancient Indian practice of health and well-being that involves holding and moving between various postures, using specified breathing methods, and achieving altering states of consciousness through meditation. While the broader aim of traditional yogic practices is unifying mind and body with spirit, in the West, it has come to be seen as a relaxing or muscle-toning physical activity depending on the yoga style.

One of the basic tenets of chronic pain is that it has both mental and physical origins and manifestations. It is a mind-body phenomenon that requires a mind-body approach. Yoga seems to be a perfect practice to relieve chronic pain. Let's discuss why this is.

One of the causes of pain is the hypertonicity (tightness) of muscles that constrict blood flow, reducing the amount of fresh oxygen and nutrients in circulation that allow toxins to accumulate in muscle tissue. Yoga is structured around the practice of physical movements that gently move the body. These movements are within the normal ranges of motion and do not require great exertion or flexibility, and will not cause sprains and tears while being performed. When the muscles are supple and the blood is moving, pain is reduced and the mental anguish and physical restrictions of that pain are diminished.

Regardless of which yoga method is practiced, studies have confirmed its healing properties. In fact, many studies have found that the regular practice of yoga can reduce blood pressure by as much as 15 mm/Hg (millimeters of mercury in blood pressure reading). With extended practice of yoga, a level of fitness is achieved and weight loss is experienced, which are also responsible for lowering of blood pressure and reduction of the effects of daily stress. Reduction of stress, lowering of blood pressure, calmness of mind, and slowed breathing are all tools that help reduce pain and symptoms of headaches and migraines.

Yoga can be an effective method for decreasing pain by its ability to induce a deep calming effect and slower breathing pattern, which assists in the relaxation of muscles and reduction of trigger points and systemic inflammation. This ancient practice brings down the stress-induced fight or flight response, thereby reducing the levels of the hormones adrenaline and cortisol that are pumping through your system.

Yoga practices, especially those with a spiritual component, also offer practitioners an emotional experience along with their physical movements, fostering feelings of love, kindness, compassion, and forgiveness. These feelings alone reduce the way people react to daily stress and the people around them. Stress causes pain, so less stress means less tension in the body and therefore less pain.

The body has learned ways of reacting to stress with protective measures like tension and pain. To overcome those ingrained responses, one needs to retrain the body's response to the mind. Practicing yoga on a weekly or bi-weekly basis has proven effective at doing this. It gives the mind and body a new pattern of relaxation and quietness. Yoga teaches one to use their mind to observe their body, to control posture, to regulate breathing ... all in an effort to allow them to take control of their experiences and how their experiences take hold in the body.

The on-going practice of yoga is transformative. It changes stress and pain responses into healing responses. Over time, it brings one to feel a sense of self-empowerment, vitality, and relaxed, stress-free living.

Pain and energy drain comes from tight muscles and tense minds. When the mind is tense, the muscles also become tense. When muscles become tense, they restrict blood flow, decrease range of motion, and can cause trigger points. Trigger points are painful dime-sized "knots" deep in the muscle tissue that can cause pain for weeks on end.

Ancient Exercises for Headache Relief

Easing mental stresses and physical muscle contractions is a must if you are striving for relief from headaches and migraines. When you are relaxed very little energy is consumed, which allows the body to recharge and repair. These periods of regeneration, just like when sleeping, are vital to proper pain-free functioning.

One natural way of relaxing both mind and body is through the regular practice of yoga. By assuming the yoga postures, known as *asanas*, one is able to relax, stretch, and tone the body at the same time. How?

Each posture is held for a period of time. This allows toning of the muscles necessary to hold the posture. However, since the postures are all designed to be assumed within the body's normal range of motion, there is little stress or strain. And with low stress, comes slow breathing that relaxes both the mind and the body. Thus, in each moment the yoga *asanas* are held, the person's mind and body relax and recharge. Just like while sleeping, but with the added benefit of gentle, strain-free toning.

When the muscles are toned, they are better able to hold the body in correct posture throughout the day. An imbalance in muscle tone or muscle suppleness is a cause of chronic body pain. If muscle A is strong and muscle B is weak, then A carries the load and B suffers injury while along for the ride. Moreover, neck pain on one side is a sign that the muscles on one side of the neck are either weaker or tenser than the muscles on the other side of the neck. Pain is the result. Yoga does wonders at reducing pain and stripping ourselves of many of the emotional and stress-based triggers of chronic headaches and migraines.

HOW TO IMPLEMENT THESE EXERCISES

It is not necessary to engage in all of these exercises to overcome your headaches and migraines. Choosing even one to begin with is a step in the right direction. Two of them are even better. I recommend beginning with QiGong standing exercises and mindful walking. These can be done at different times of the day without cutting into your daily schedule – you can stand watching the news, waiting in line or talking to friends, and as you walk everywhere. If you can join a class that offers yoga or Tai Chi, then these can be added to your routine, too. Some people like the solitary time in walking and standing, while others enjoy the group dynamic and support that yoga and Tai Chi classes can offer. Each of them is good and offers similar results if done correctly. So go ahead and start moving with some safe and low-impact mind–body exercises. They are another of the important pieces in the puzzle of relief from headaches and migraines.

CHAPTER REVIEW

- Make exercise a part of your headache relief program, despite the myths to the contrary.
- I suggest effective mind-body programs like Mindful Walking, QiGong, Tai Chi, and Yoga because they are easier to practice in spite of the constant stiffness, inflammation, and pain that accompany headaches.
- Beyond the general health benefits of these exercises, these particular programs help focus your thoughts, emotions, and spirit – reducing stress and anxiety that often comes with chronic headaches and migraines.
- Start by choosing one of these programs – it is an important step in the right direction.

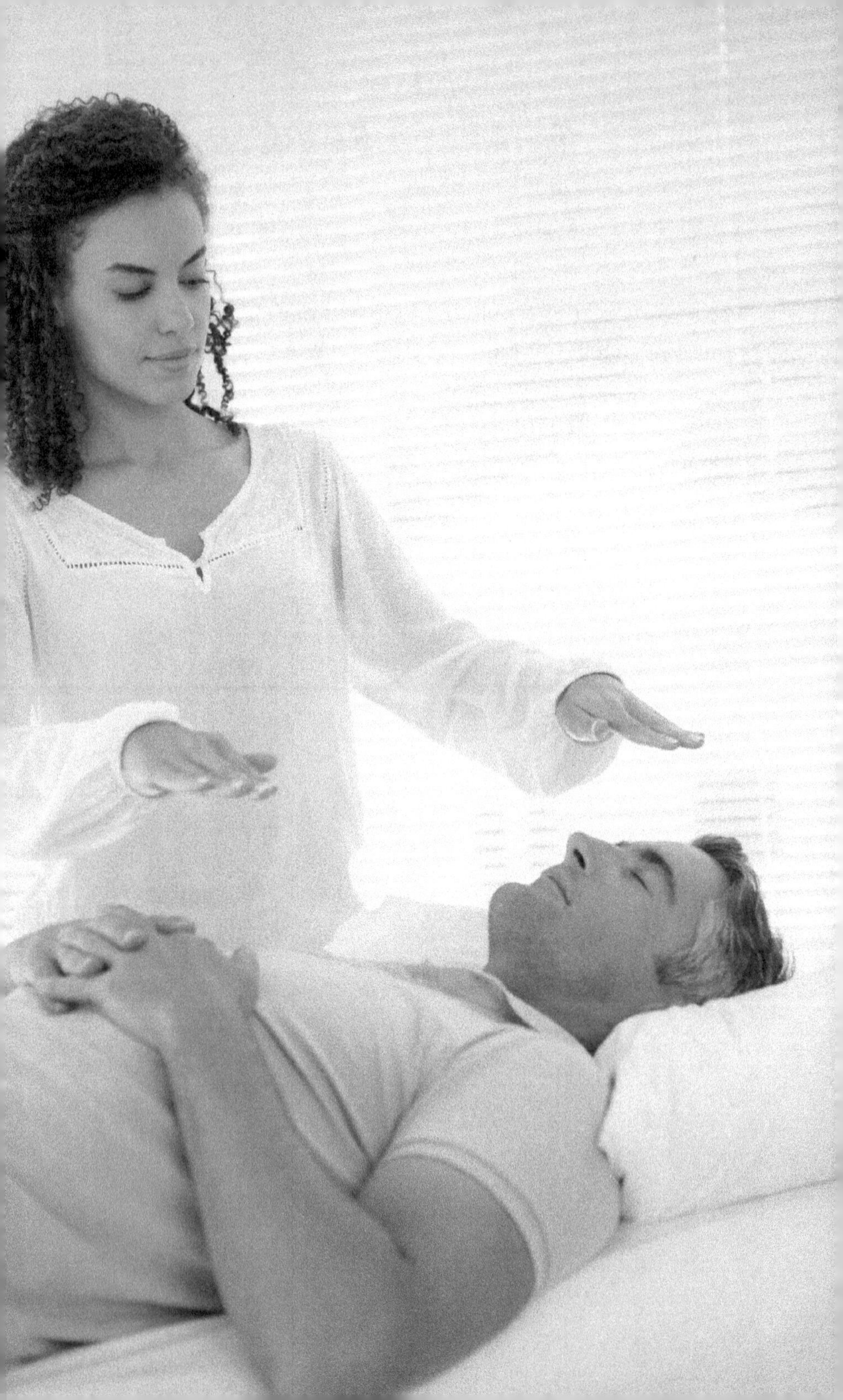

CHAPTER 17

ENERGY MEDICINE FOR HEADACHE RELIEF

Everything in the Universe is made up of energy and is vibrating at specific frequencies. There are high frequencies and low frequencies. The human body is a physical body constructed of energetic vibrations—the constant movement of protons, electrons, neutrons, atoms, and molecules.

All aspects of health and well-being – especially pain – are tied to energetic frequencies. The problem is, most of us who suffer chronic pain only get the "pain channel" and keep ourselves "tuned in" to it 24/7. Thus the "pain frequency" is maintained and our suffering needlessly prolonged.

If you tune in to an opera channel on your radio, you will get opera, not country music. If you dial your mother on the cell phone, you won't get cousin Betty. If you say bad things about people, you will lose friends. "You reap what you sow," is a good example of the power of attraction, the power of like energy meeting like energy.

If your mental energy is vibrating at a low frequency, you will have trouble studying, thinking, or remembering names, places or events. If your physical energy is blocked or sluggish, you will experience aches and pains such as sciatica, headache, fibromyalgia, and others. In short, low frequency = low function and poor health; high frequency = high functioning and good health.

You must change your energetic frequency to feel better and live better.

THE ENERGY BODY

Traditional cultures around the world built their healing models on correcting energetic imbalances in the body. The role of Shamans in Siberia, Alaska, and Southeast Asia was to eradicate "bad spirits" (i.e., negative energy) from the body to restore physical or mental health in those suffering. The entire pantheon of Chinese and Indian healing practices was built on the premise of energy systems and pathways in the body that, when blocked, cause pain and disease. Clearing these channels or centers of blocked energy (e.g., toxins, spasms) is what restores health to the ill and offers relief to the pain sufferer.

Perhaps the most common term used to talk about human energy is aura. This is a general term used to describe the color, mood or quality of five overlapping energy layers. These layers of energy (or energy bodies) refer to the spiritual, mental, emotional, etheric, and physical energies that make up humans.

Energy is developed, stored, and moved in the body through the adrenals, organs, chakra centers, and meridian pathways. There is a saying in Traditional Chinese Medicine (TCM) that explains why we experience pain: "Where there is energy blockage, there is pain. Where energy moves freely, there is no pain." This is based on "The Three Hidden Imbalances that Cause Headaches" outlined in Chapter 7.

The key to pain relief and lasting health, then, is to open the energy channels, raise your vibration frequency, and keep your energy moving at all times. There are a number of alternative therapies whose primary function is just that.

POLARITY THERAPY

Like other energy medicine methodologies, polarity therapy sees the human body as comprising "life energy." However, polarity therapy takes the view that the energy body is in a state of constant "pulsation," with positive and negative poles and a neutral position. These poles and position form a kind of energetic "template" along the body, on which a practitioner can apply touch and pressure to alter the pulsations and derive pain relief and improve general states of health.

While it shares common ideas with acupressure and QiGong, polarity therapy is more aligned with Indian Ayurvedic medicine and modern osteopathic and chiropractic theories of the body. When people have gone through the complete series of acupuncture or QiGong treatments recommended by their practitioner, and have not found substantial relief, polarity therapy may be the next best modality to embrace. Oftentimes, a person's polarity (positive/negative energy poles) is reversed, and one or more polarity sessions can correct this.

QUANTUM TOUCH®

The new kid on the block, in terms of hands-on energy work, is called Quantum Touch.® It is both a method for individuals to work on themselves and for practitioners to work on those in need of its healing potential. It does this using simple methods where life force energy is amplified and entrained. This process helps the body facilitate its own healing process.

The claims that Quantum Touch® relieves chronic pain was put to the test through an eight-week pilot study in which the investigators used 12 volunteer adult patients (men and women ages 18 to 64) who were randomly selected and randomly assigned to an experimental and control group of six volunteers in each group. Both groups were blindfolded and received hands-on touch; however, only the experimental group was given the Quantum Touch® energy. What was made very clear through the research was that Quantum Touch® healing is effective and has a positive impact on clients in the area of chronic musculoskeletal pain. This holistic modality, like others before it, can now offer itself to the world of health and wellness as a viable method of pain management with documented evidence of its impact and effectiveness.

REIKI

Reiki is a Japanese energy technique for reducing stress and inducing relaxation to help promote the free-flow of energy in the body. Reiki is both a non-touch and a "laying on of hands" by a practitioner for its benefits to be gained.

Reiki practitioners place their hands on patients in various configurations that are modeled on ancient Tibetan and Chinese powerful healing symbols. It is believed that re-creating these symbols on the body will allow "God's energy" to flow from the Universe through the practitioner and into the patient. This energy, which is vibrating at a high frequency, will lift the low energy of the sufferer to relieve pain and illness.

Reiki has become a popular healing modality among nurses in hospitals. The patient does not have to be awake for them to administer a few minutes of healing touch. It may be the easiest of all the energy healing systems to find a practitioner and also feels really good. However, of all the methods I have personally studied and been treated with, Reiki seems to have the least corrective benefits. Good for relaxation and acute symptomatic relief, but not as effective for long-term relief based on being a truly corrective body therapy.

QIGONG THERAPY

QiGong refers to specific health exercises or techniques for regulating the body, mind, and breath. They involve visualization, movement, posture and self-massage to effect interior balance and thus positive changes in health.

Regular practice of QiGong aids in regulating the functions of the central nervous system. Along with exercising and controlling one's mind and body, QiGong influences one's physical states and pathological conditions. Concurrently, the practice of QiGong emits latent energy within the human body, enabling the practitioner to use them to their fullest potential. Regular practice increases the body's ability to adapt to and defend against the natural/physical environment in which we live.

The primary use of QiGong today is to improve one's health, thus extending life. This is known as "medical" or "healing" QiGong of which there are three subdivisions:

1) Applied clinical therapy, whereby a Chinese doctor emits (projects) his own qi into a patient's body to affect a cure;

2) Self-regulating exercises, whereby a person chooses a QiGong program and practices the exercises over a period of at least 100 days to improve his or her own health;

3) A combination of clinical QiGong treatments from a doctor and an individual's personal self-regulating QiGong training program. Within the self-practice method, exercises are done in any combination of three ways: static postures, slow movements, meditation, and breathing exercises.

ACUPUNCTURE

For thousands of years, the Chinese have been using a unique method of health maintenance called acupuncture. Today, acupuncture is a household word and part of America's out-of-pocket healthcare toolbox. But this ancient needle-and-channel therapy remains an outlier when it comes to acceptance in the mainstream medical establishment. However, a pair of studies coming out of Duke University shed positive light on the benefits of acupuncture over drugs for pain relief, and represents an important step toward giving acupuncture more Western credibility.

In one report, researchers at Duke performed a meta-analysis of 31 clinical studies involving some 4,000 patients on the effects of acupuncture for headache relief compared to treatment with medication. Their findings: "Acupuncture is more effective than medication in reducing the severity and frequency of chronic headaches."[1]

When comparing the data, the researchers found that 62% of those given acupuncture for headaches reported pain relief. Only 45% of those taking medication for their head pain reported relief. Two important points to take note of: 1) The studies were conducted on people suffering various types of headaches (tension, migraine, etc.), and, 2) proper acupuncture point prescription was essential.

Acupuncture stimulates different points in the body that fall along energy lines called meridians. Depending on the location of the headache (top of head, side of head) and the type of symptoms associated with the pain (throbbing, burning, sweating), the practitioner alters the points being stimulated by the acupuncture needles. Consequently, the acupuncture is used differently for different headache types and locations. It is, therefore, more specific. However, the theory on which the therapy is based remains unchanged: Where there is a blockage of energy in the body, there is pain. Release the blockage; diminish the pain. And while several studies seem to show that sham acupuncture (using non-specific points) offers some relief, the Duke study found that the greatest relief of pain is gained from using correct needle technique administered to the correct acu-points.

"One of the barriers to treatment with acupuncture," says Dr. Tong Joo Gan, the study lead, "is getting people to understand that while needles are used, it is not a painful experience. It is a method for releasing your body's own natural painkillers." Gan is correct. In fact, the needles used in acupuncture are so thin that they can be tied into a knot with two fingers. Those who fear the pain associated with the hypodermic needles used in medical shots are reassured to know that 20 acupuncture needles can fit into the opening of the standard medical needle. Acupuncture needles are so thin, in fact, that you can insert one of these needles into an inflated balloon and the balloon does not pop.

FREQUENCY SPECIFIC MICROCURRENT (FSM) THERAPY

Frequency specific microcurrent (FSM) therapy specifically treats myofacial neuropathic pain that reduces inflammatory cytokines (polypeptide regulators). In other words, it helps reduce trigger points and fascial constrictions that cause pain, which include sensations like "pins and needles," coldness or burning, and numbness or itching caused by a damaged or diseased sensory system, as is common in migraines.

FSM is a non-invasive therapy that requires the use of a two-channel micro amperage current device, which can be purchased online. The treatment requires two separate channels of voltage (13Hz and 396Hz) to be connected to the patient while attempting to move their affected limbs to their utmost range of motion. Clinical studies show that these specific frequencies, when used simultaneously, can effectively treat nerve and muscle pain, reduce inflammation, and clear scar tissue. Other frequencies help reduce the pain associated with kidney stones, and aid in healing of asthma, liver dysfunction, irritable bowel syndrome (IBS), and other conditions.

PULSED ELECTROMAGNETIC FREQUENCY (PEMF) THERAPY

For many, the idea that electromagnetic frequency (EMF) smog is harmful has never crossed their minds. If you cannot see it, it does not exist. Right? Wrong. This smog is all around us—every day, everywhere we go. It originates from the frequencies of cell towers, Wi-Fi in cafes, cell and cordless phones, high-definition (HD) televisions, laptop computers, microwaves, and especially in our vehicles. EMFs are making us ill and killing us slowly by breaking down the very structure of our cells. There is no escaping it.

Martin Blank, Ph.D. of Columbia University says, "Cells in the body react to low level EMFs and produce a biochemical stress response. Our safety standards are inadequate. People need to sit up and pay attention."[2]

We are immersed in a sea of EMF radiation. It comes from cordless phones and base stations, cell phones and towers, electrical appliances, computers, fluorescent lighting, Bluetooth devices, Wi-Fi installations, and more than 2,000 satellites for GPS and TV and radio communications.

"New research is suggesting that nearly all of the human plagues, which emerged in the 20th century, including leukemia in children, female breast cancer, malignant melanomas, immune system disorders, asthma and others, can be tied in some way to our use of electricity."

Here's a breakdown of the negative health effects of prolonged EMF exposure. That is, exposure over a scant two milligauss:

- Interferes with our body's intracellular communications and cell membrane function.
- Reduces hemoglobin surface area and interferes with blood's ability to carry oxygen and nutrients into our cells and take waste products out.
- Activates proto-oncogenes (which can cause cancer).
- Increases permeability of the blood-brain barrier and affects intra-cerebral pressure, which some believe seems to bring on Alzheimer's, Parkinson's, autism, multiple sclerosis and other neurodegenerative disorders.
- Causes DNA breaks and chromosome aberrations.
- Increases free radical production.
- Causes cell stress and premature aging.
- Causes changes in brain function, including memory loss, learning impairment, headaches and fatigue.

- Reduces melatonin secretion. Melatonin is responsible for sleep patterns and helps protect the body against cancer, among other things.

- Causes many microorganisms living in the human body to generate increased levels of their own toxins, affecting people's health in a myriad way.

In a nutshell, each of our cells is surrounded by something called a phospholipid bi-layer membrane, commonly known as the cell membrane. Embedded in the cell membrane are numerous proteins that act as receptors for various molecules, including enzymes. These receptors translate the positive-negative signals on the cell's exterior into its interior, and these signals then trigger various biological processes.

When we're affected by external electromagnetic fields, the high-speed positive-negative polarity switching within these fields, from hundreds to millions of times per second, interferes with our cells' internal signaling process. Basically, it confuses them and causes them to become paralyzed.

A product recently permitted into the United States claims it can reverse this damage in only eight minutes, two to three times a day. It's called the MRS2000, and it is a German-engineered medical device that uses pulsed, healthy EMFs to counter the debilitating effects of today's EMF smog and help bring people to optimal health.

It turns out (much like the discovery of both good and bad cholesterol), that certain EMFs are actually good for us. In fact, we can't live without them. As a result, much research has gone into refining pulsed EMF therapy and the results are impressive.

Paul Rosch, M.D., of New York Medical College, went on record to say, "While EMFs are responsible for quite a bit of damage, don't throw the baby out with the bathwater. Pulsed electromagnetic frequency (PEMF) therapies have been shown to be beneficial for stress related disorders, anxiety, insomnia, arthritis, depression, and more. They also may be safer and more effective than drugs."

Thousands of clinical studies are proving its value, and PEMF therapy is beginning to get the recognition it deserves. While experts may not all agree on what EMF exposure levels cause which health issues, the lack of evidence out there suggests we would be foolish not to apply the precautionary principle and reduce our exposure. Using the MRS2000 could be a big step in the right direction.

CEFALY DEVICE STIMULATES AWAY HEADACHES

Stimulation on the skin surface has been an integral part of various therapies since the beginning of time. Recently, the Food and Drug Administration (FDA) approved the first ever use of an electro-stim device to help combat chronic headaches. And it looks like this is an effective therapy.

How Electrical Stimulation Works

Applying an electrical current to stimulate the nerves on the skin surface is known by several names, including transcutaneous electrical nerve stimulation, electro-stim, micro current therapy, and neuro-stimulation (among others). An electrical charge is applied to the skin via conductive pads, acupuncture needles, nerve conduction devices and other means. An electrical impulse, which depolarizes nerve fibers, is sent to the skin. This current temporarily blocks pain signals through application of the therapeutic electrical signal from the device. Devices like these are commonly used in acupuncture clinics, physical therapy centers, and chiropractic practices. Mostly, such devices have been used to reduce pain associated with neck, back, and limbs. Recently, however, the FDA also approved the first-ever stimulation unit used to specifically treat migraine headaches.

The Belgian-made device, known as Cefaly, has been proven effective in clinical trials for more than half of all migraine sufferers, and is also approved for pain prevention of any type. The Cefaly device is connected to specific areas of the forehead with adhesive electrodes. These target the impulses of the trigeminal nerve, a nerve that travels from the neck and wraps up and around the head. While the exact cause of migraines has been uncertain (although triggers are identified), these specific headaches are thought to be related both to vasoconstriction and trigeminal nerve function.

Clinical Studies Show Positive Results

Several studies over the past few years have yielded some strong results. In 2011, the journal *BMC Neurology* published the findings of a double-blind versus placebo study on the sedative effects of the Cefaly's suborbital transcutaneous neurostimulation (sTNS).[3] For the study, 30 healthy subjects underwent a series of four vigilance tests carried out under four different experimental conditions: wit1) Without the presence of the neuro-stimulation device; 2) With sham supraorbital TNS; 3) With low-frequency supraorbital TNS; and, 4) With high-frequency supraorbital TNS. There was found to be a "statistically significant ($p < 0.001$) decrease in vigilance (insomnia) and attention during high-frequency TNS, while there were no changes during the other experimental conditions," leading researchers to conclude that "supraorbital high frequency TNS applied with the Cefaly® device decreases vigilance in healthy volunteers."

A 2013 double-blind, randomized, sham-controlled trial on the effectiveness of Cefaly at preventing migraines, was published in the journal *Neurology*. The trials were conducted at five Belgian tertiary headache clinics where patients who suffered at least two migraines monthly were given sham or actual stimulator for 20 minutes daily over a three-month period. The results showed a change in the numbers of days with migraine per month in 50% of responders. The results: "The therapeutic gain (26%) is within the range of those reported for other preventive drug and non-drug anti-migraine treatments. This study provides Class III evidence that treatment with a supraorbital transcutaneous stimulator is effective and safe as a preventive therapy for migraine."

A 2013 cohort study of 2,313 headache sufferers, testing the effectiveness of the Cefaly device against migraine, was published in the *Journal of Headache and Pain*.[4] The study responders used the devise in home for a testing period of 40 days after which 54.4% of study subjects were satisfied with the devise and willing to purchase one of their own. The study showed the TNS device to be superior to sham stimulation.

The Cefaly device is safe, gentle, and simple to use. It is also non-invasive and does not damage the liver or kidneys. Also, by using this device to help reduce the onset and pain associated with migraine, patients may be able to reduce the frequency and amount of prescription medication they may currently be taking. Currently, the device is available through prescription only. If you suffer intractable migraines, have a talk with your healthcare provider and see if this new treatment is another answer in your migraine-fighting toolbox.

CERENA TMS DEVICE

According to their press release in December of 2013 the U.S. FDA allowed marketing of the Cerena Transcranial Magnetic Stimulator (TMS), the first device to relieve pain caused by migraine headaches that are preceded by an aura (a visual, sensory or motor disturbance immediately preceding the onset of a migraine attack).[5]

"Millions of people suffer from migraines and this new device represents a new treatment option for some patients," said Christy Foreman, director of the Office of Device Evaluation in the FDA's Center for Devices and Radiological Health.

The Cerena TMS is a prescription device used after the onset of pain associated with migraine headaches preceded by an aura. Using both hands to hold the device against the back of the head, the user presses a button to release a pulse of magnetic energy to stimulate the occipital cortex in the brain, which may stop or lessen the pain associated with migraine headaches preceded by an aura.

The FDA reviewed a randomized control clinical trial of 201 patients who had mostly moderate to strong migraine headaches and who had auras preceding at least 30% of their migraines. Of the study subjects, 113 recorded treating a migraine at least once when pain was present. Analysis of these 113 subjects was used to support marketing authorization of the Cerena TMS for the acute treatment of pain associated with migraine headache with aura.

The study showed that nearly 38% of subjects who used the Cerena TMS when they had migraine pain were pain-free two hours after using the device compared to about 17% of patients in the control group. After 24 hours, nearly 34% of the Cerena TMS users were pain-free compared to 10% in the control group.

CHAPTER REVIEW

- The entire Universe, including the human body, is made of energy, vibrating at specific frequencies.
- All aspects of health and well-being – including pain – are tied to energetic frequencies
- Unfortunately, those in chronic pain are "tuned in" to the "pain channel," keeping themselves focused solely on their pain, and resonating at a "pain frequency."
- You can and must change your energetic frequency to feel better and live better.
- You can shift your energy with practices and methods like: Polarity Therapy, Quantum Touch, Reiki, QiGong Therapy, Acupuncture, FSM Therapy, PEMF Therapy, and the new Cefaly and Cerena TMS devices.

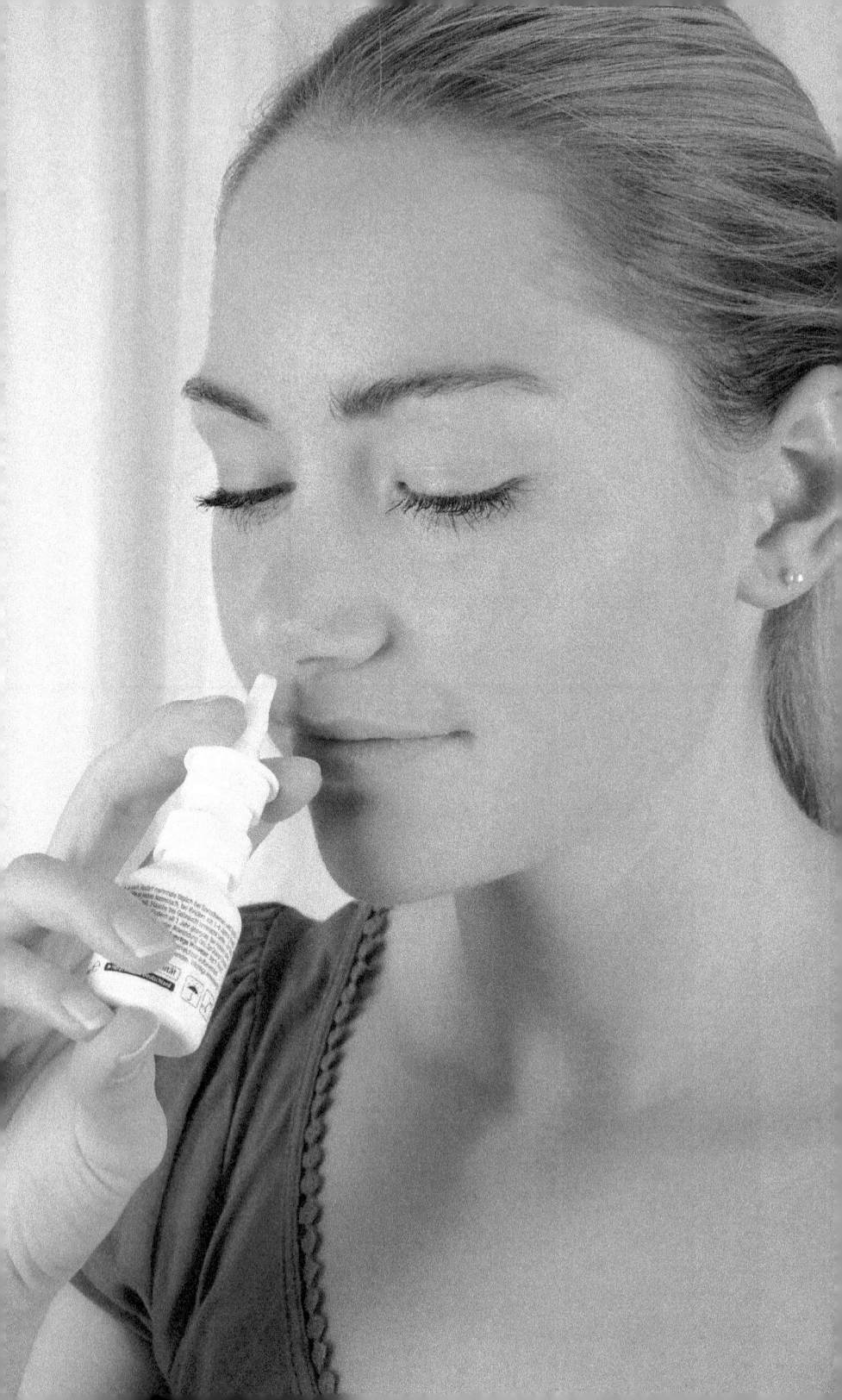

CHAPTER 18

UNUSUAL INTERVENTIONS FOR HEADACHE RELIEF

The previous chapters in this section have shared some proven and powerful methods for balancing the body to reduce and prevent headaches and migraines. But there are even more ways available, with new research shining light on the efficacy of natural and alternative methods for headache relief. So this chapter presents a handful of more solutions that can help you on your path to a headache-free life, including: topical analgesics, migraine sprays, green light therapy and cannabis. Let's take a look.

TOPICAL PRODUCTS FOR PAIN AND INFLAMMATION

When searching for relief from headache pain associated with inflammation, swelling and stiffness, applying topical creams or ointments can provide some good, short-term relief. These products are found in abundance in American drugstores and in Asian markets. Though the Eastern and Western versions of these products have some different ingredients, they serve the same purpose: Instant relief for acute symptoms of headaches, including muscle tightness, neck pain, and reduced blood flow.

Topical pain products are mostly used for short-term relief, as once their active ingredients have metabolized in the body, their value is greatly diminished. For effectiveness over the long term they should be applied three times per day, and as a part of the overall Headache Relief Action Plan.

How Topical Products Work

There are several key ways in which the various topical products help reduce pain, swelling, inflammation, and stiffness. Many of the products are known as counter-irritants. This is a fancy way of saying they irritate your skin in some way to shift your mind and nervous system off the pressing issue. In other words, ingredients like menthol, wintergreen oil, and eucalyptus are used to counter the symptomatic irritant by creating a new irritant, like redness or sensations of cool or warmth on the skin.

This process is also known as "gate control" or "gating," as it gates off or blocks the receptors in the skin from sending pain signals to the brain, instead sending the heat or cooling signal. This then "tricks" the mind to focus on the new irritant, and tricks the nervous system into think the area is hot (to send more blood) or cold (to send more heat) and, thus, improve the original, bothersome symptoms.

Many of the topical products contain salicylates, which is a class of chemicals that acts in a way similar to NSAIDs. In other words, they have topical analgesic (pain reducing) and anti-inflammatory (inflammation reducing) qualities. These chemicals occur in nature in mint, menthol, and peppermint, for example. They work by inhibiting the synthesis of prostaglandin, the naturally occurring and chemically related fatty acids that aid in blood pressure and body temperature regulation and control inflammation and vascular permeability. Like NSAIDs, they can be useful in reducing pain and inflammation in the shoulders, neck, and temples that trigger headaches.

Ingredients and Best Usage

Many of the most popular pain-relieving creams and gels share common ingredients. If you look at the product labels, you will likely see one or more of the following active ingredients, among others: Wintergreen, camphor, menthol, capsaicin, and salicylate.

In terms of best way to apply and use the products, please read the labels of any of the products you are going to use prior to applying them to your body. Many are harmful if applied to open wounds and scratches, if they touch the eyes or are accidentally ingested. Make sure you know the possible negative effects and have a plan for washing the affected area or otherwise in case of ingestion, etc.

These products are made more powerful (or at least felt more) when applied right before or after a workout or hot shower, as the skin pores and blood vessels are expanded and can absorb more of the product quickly. However, be warned that this may be too much to handle. If the product brings a heat sensation, it will be increased many fold and may be unbearable. Also, be sure to wash your hands immediately after application to prevent accidental touching of your eyes, face, mouth, or private areas.

Part of maintaining an effective wellness program, like "The Headache Relief Action Plan," is to have realistic expectations. Keep in mind that while effective at reducing acute symptoms like pain and inflammation, topical products often take around two months to have longer-lasting effects. You should look to them as supporting symptomatic relief in the moment, while working on your lifestyle changes and therapies to make longer and deeper changes.

SPRAY AWAY MIGRAINE PAIN

Dr. Kenneth Mandato and associates at the Albany Medical Center in Albany, NY, have come a long way to helping relieve migraine pain, severity, and occurrence. They've discovered a minimally invasive treatment using a type of "migraine spray."[1] As you're reading this, they will have just presented the findings of their independent study at the annual meeting of the Society of Interventional Radiology in Atlanta, GA.

The first thing I noticed is that the study for migraine reduction and prevention was not done by neurologists or by Big Pharma. Dr. Mandato and his team of radiologist partners carried it out. Their new procedure "significantly alleviates" the pain associated with migraines. It works very simply and non-invasively by spraying a local anesthetic called Lidocaine (Xylocaine) directly on the nerves located inside the nasal cavity.

To administer the Lidocaine solution, researchers inserted a small catheter into the nasal passages of each of the 112 patient participants. All 112 participants were previously identified as being affected by cluster headaches and their migraine symptoms and pain levels were assessed.

Researchers delivered a dose of the solution to the cluster of nerves located at the back of the nasal cavity, known as the Meckel's ganglion. There nerves are associated with the trigeminal nerve, which is now believed to be largely associated with headaches, both general and migraine. The researchers believe that the Lidocaine somehow "short-circuits this neural highway's pathway associated with recurrent headaches or migraines."

It must work, because a single treatment reduced pain levels of a migraine episode from a self-reported 8 (out of 10) to a 4 (out of 10). What's more, the 35% pain reduction lasted a full month after the treatment. In fact, 94% of the people in the study found fast and lasting pain relief, which is a very strong indicator of good things to come.

If you've ever needed to have an analgesic injection for migraines, then the news most promising about this treatment is that you won't have to worry anymore about toxicity that can harm the liver, kidneys, and GI tract.

And at some point, you might be able to have a spray bottle that you use maybe twice a year, and carry with you for emergencies. I look forward to more tests and peer review. We need to see the long-term effects to the nerves as a result of the direct Lidocaine application. I'll be keeping an eye out and will update you as I learn more.

GREEN LIGHT THERAPY FOR PHOTOPHOBIA

One of the hallmarks of classic migraine is the pre-headache aura that affects 80% of sufferers. There is also a severe sensitivity to light (known as photophobia) once a migraine or cluster headaches is in full swing. When I would get these headaches, I'd have to lie down in a dark room with a light pillow or towel covering my eyes. And in addition to the nausea and pain, this light issue made doing anything at all except lying still in the dark an impossible dream.

Well, another new remedy is forthcoming that promises good results with photophobia. Researchers from Harvard Medical School found that headaches can be relieved by as much as 20% and the symptoms of photophobia can be eased with a narrow band of green light.[2]

Harvard Medical School researchers at Beth Israel Deaconess Medical Center have found that exposing migraine sufferers to a narrow band of green light significantly reduces photophobia and can reduce headache severity. Their study was published in the journal *Brain*.[3] The downside is that the bulb they use is prohibitively expensive and thus out of reach for most people. In the meantime, you can keep an eye out for more on this, and other green-light therapies that may show up in your searches. Green light therapy seems promising for this symptom of migraine.

NATURE'S "WEED" HELPFUL FOR MIGRAINES

It's funny how things change. What was once considered the lore of the lazy, the herb of fringe spirituality, and a schedule 1 controlled substance that is federally illegal is now looked at by many as a miracle cure for all ailments. I'm talking about cannabis.

Over the past decade, and especially the past few of years, the rhetoric around marijuana use has changed. The pot-smoking camp has turned and pushed toward cannabis as panacea. And of course proponents of medical marijuana who claim cannabis cures everything from cancer to migraines, from multiple sclerosis to Crohn's disease, will tell you that the NIH and FDA, in the pockets of Big Pharma, are keeping it illegal so they and they alone can extract its essence, patent it, and sell it as a prescription drug.

I read an article on marijuana and migraine headache that quoted a study from the journal *Pharmacotherapy*:

> *"It turns out some patients diagnosed with migraine headaches saw a significant drop in their frequency when treated with medical marijuana. On average, the number of migraines dropped from 10.4 to 4.6 headaches per month—a number*

considered statistically and clinically significant for migraine sufferers...Scientists say marijuana has anti-inflammatory and pain-relieving properties. It also triggers the release of serotonin and dopamine—neurotransmitters that cause feelings of happiness. These characteristics make it an ideal way to combat migraine headaches."[4]

A bit more research showed that state-by-state marijuana is becoming increasingly more legal. In some places, only the medicinal CBD components are legal, but only if you are a legal resident of the given state and have a prescription from your doctor. In other places, the recreational THC components are legal. A good website that provides a broad overview about the laws, legality and a video of President Obama discussing cannabis is found here.[5]

Currently, four states have legalized the recreational use of marijuana: Alaska, Colorado, Oregon, Washington, and the District of Columbia. However, 24 states have made legal the medicinal use of cannabis: Alaska, Arizona, California, Colorado, Connecticut, Delaware, Hawaii, Illinois, Maine, Maryland, Massachusetts, Michigan, Minnesota, Montana, Nevada, New Hampshire, New Jersey, New Mexico, New York, Oregon, Pennsylvania, Rhode Island, Vermont, and Washington.

So if your headaches are intractable and you are open-minded about the potential effect that medical marijuana may have for you, check your state laws or make a trip to a legal state and see how you feel.

CHAPTER REVIEW

- While we are all the same in many way, we also are different. The interventions that may help one person may do nothing for another. So many factors are involved, which is why "The Headache Relief Action Plan" is such a holistic, broad, multi-disciplinary program for prevention.

- When you have tried many interventions and feel you are at a plateau and want to try something different or new, look to the topical creams, green light therapy, migraine spray, and cannabis options. They can help with short-term relief of symptoms and help get you through a bad headache, while you re-align your lifestyle in favor of headache prevention.

CHAPTER 19

PAIN RELIEF INTERVENTIONS FOR SPECIFIC HEADACHE LOCATIONS

The success of the DIY, self-cure approach of "The Headache Relief Action Plan" is identifying WHERE you first feel the onset of the headache... and taking immediate steps to stop the headache-in-progress, and make long-term, lifestyle changes to prevent headaches from triggering again.

PROBLEMS WITH HEADACHE DEFINITIONS

Headache sufferers are told they have migraines, cluster headaches, tension headaches, or any number of other headache types. Then they are prescribed medication to help relieve the pain, such as Imitrex for migraines. The problem is, using headache name definitions to base treatment can become a losing proposition. Why?

Because most people get more than one kind of headache. It is not uncommon for people who suffer stress headaches or sinus headaches to also experience migraine headaches or sleep-deprivation headaches. And so just because one might suffer "migraines" does not mean the headache they get on a given day is a migraine. Therefore, the migraine medication should not be taken for that headache.

What's more, did you know that many over-the-counter medicines marketed as "migraine relief" and "tension headache relief" actually contain the same ingredients? They are the same product being marketed and sold for different "definitions" of headaches.

GENERAL INTERVENTION TECHNIQUE

If you fall off the wagon and a headache takes hold, I highly recommend you call in late for work or leave early—depending on when the pain arises—and go through the following *Intervention Technique* to greatly diminish or entirely remove the pain and allow you to return to your normal routine—without swallowing a pain killer. It is a simple sequence of things to do that, if done at the onset of the headache, will "cancel out" the triggers before they are able to truly take hold in the body and wreak havoc. It is a sequence that combines elements of the eight-part program of headache prevention, but in a condensed and effective "quick fix" mode.

The technique sequence should bring lasting relief within 30 minutes to an hour. Here's the seven-part sequence:

- Drink three 12-ounce bottles of spring or purified water in one sitting. While you may find it difficult to do so, try your best to drink all three bottles within five minutes. This will help hydrate and detoxify the body.

Pain Relief Interventions for Specific Headache Locations

- Breathe deeply and slowly while pressing and/or massaging the following acupressure points on the body: 1) The space between the big toe and second toe; 2) the webbing between the index finger and thumb; 3) the "third eye" or forehead location between the eyebrows; 4) the temples; 5) the ear lobes; and, 6) the base of the skull. This sequence will help reduce symptoms related to stress and organ functions.

- Submerge your hands or feet in very hot water, as hot as you can stand it without burning yourself. This will draw blood away from the head and toward the hands, thereby reducing some of the vascular dilation and, by extension, the throbbing in the temporal arteries.

- Administer yourself a water enema as directed on the package. Evacuate your bowels and bladder.

- Take a therapy shower, which means no soap or shampoo (they can be toxic). Stand under the showerhead and allow the water to pour directly over your head and shoulders. Begin with very hot water and after five or more minutes, change it to cold water for a time. Return again to hot water and then reduce the water to body temperature, which is the temperature where you can barely feel the water because it matches the temperature of your own body. The combination of the hot water hand soak and this hot/cold/hot/body temperature shower will stabilize the blood vessels, which may have been constricting and dilating.

- Put on loose fitting clothes that will not obstruct breathing, lie down, and engage in cyclical breathing (four counts in and eight counts out) followed by progressive relaxation or mindfulness meditation, as you feel is needed.

- Drifting off to sleep for even 10 minutes will also help, especially if the headache was in part brought on by sleep deprivation or stress.

This sequence takes between 30 minutes to one hour to complete, but it is necessary to perform all measures in an effort to abort the single-type or mixed headache in progress *before* it has had a chance to really take hold in your body. It will work if you *allow* it to work by relaxing and letting each part do its job. If you are worried about getting someplace fast or try to force the technique, it will only add stress, anxiety, belabored breathing, irritation, and confound the headache onset in progress. However, if you follow the sequence and give yourself the time necessary to complete it, you will not further aggravate the situation or reintroduce toxins into your system, and you will be able to get on with the day with much less of a headache or none at all.

ACUPRESSURE POINTS FOR RELIEF

The next section outlines four specific areas of the head where headaches strike. Along with these are specific interventions, like the one above, that are directed toward headaches in these specific locations. Part of the process to relief is to press on acu-points for 30 seconds at a time. Most often, these points are not in the location of the headache, but found along the hands and feet or legs. Here are the point location directions and images so you can easily locate them to implement the interventions outlined below.

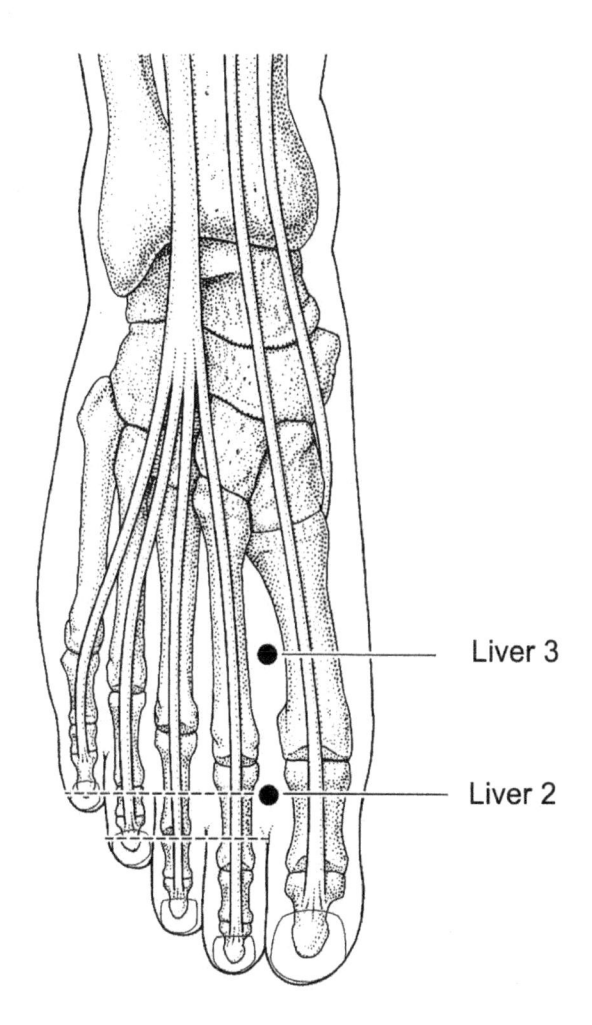

Pain Relief Interventions for Specific Headache Locations

Liver Acu-Points

Liver-2: On the dorsum of the foot between the first and second toe, near the margin of the web.

Liver-3: On the top of the foot, in the depression near the junction of the first and second metatarsal bones.

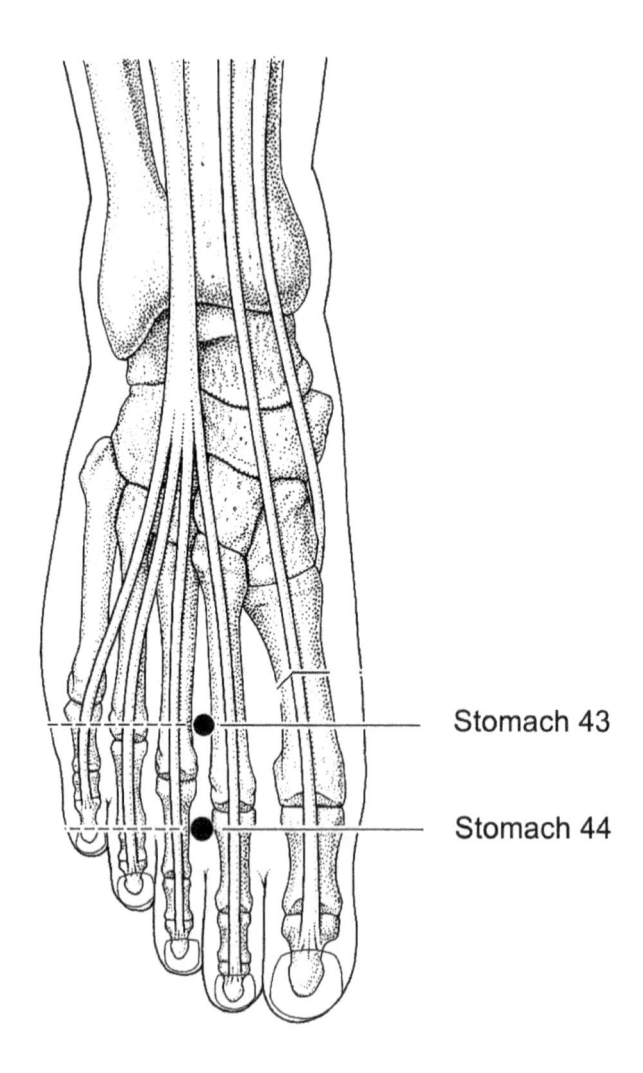

Stomach 43

Stomach 44

Stomach Acu-Points

Stomach-43: In the depression next to the junction of the second and third metatarsal bones.

Stomach-44: Near the web margin between the second and third toes, in the depression next to the second metatarso-digital joint.

Pain Relief Interventions for Specific Headache Locations

[Galbladder 34]

[Gallbladder 43]

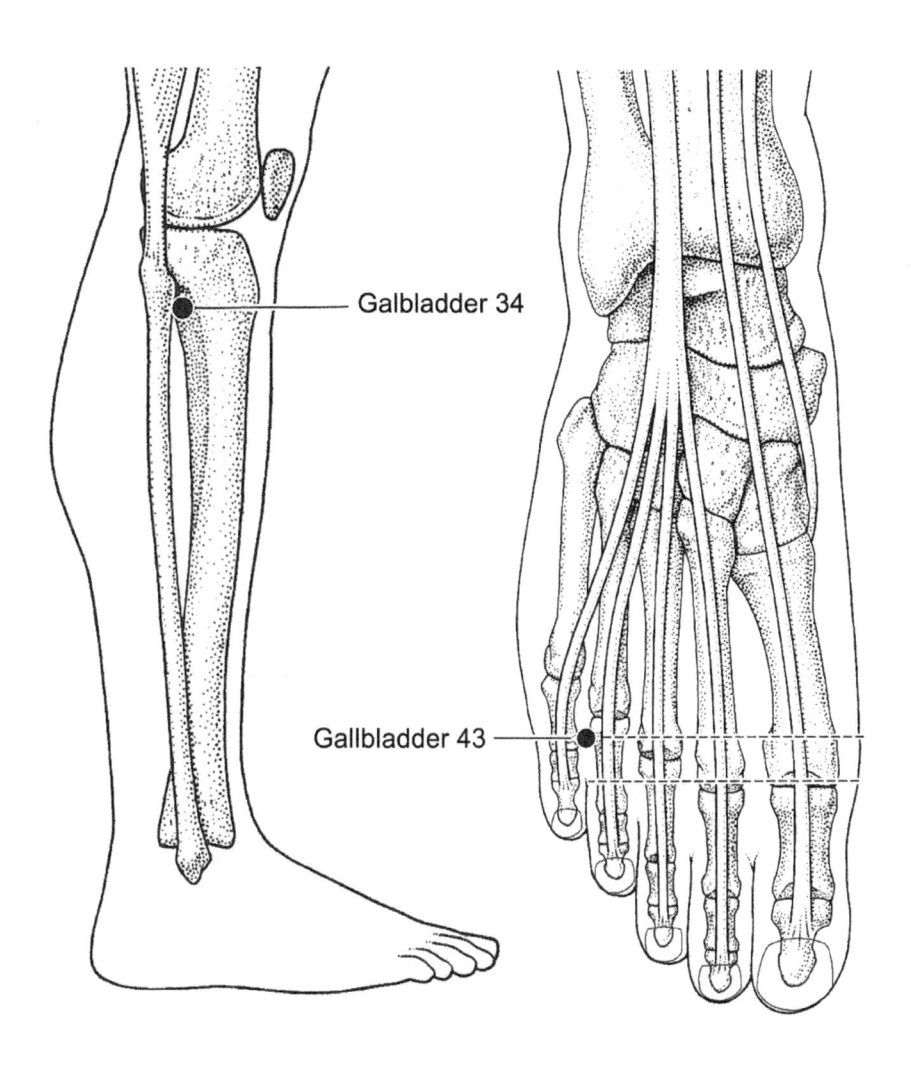

Gallbladder Acu-Points

Gallbladder-34: In the depression behind and below the head of the fibula.

Gallbladder-43: On top of the foot between the fourth and fifth toe, near the margin of the web.

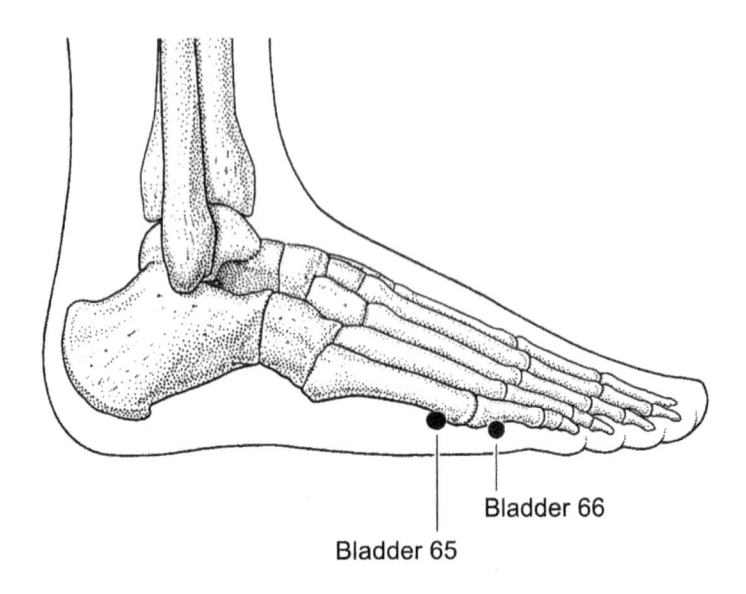

Bladder Acu-Points

Bladder-65: Below the head of the fifth metatarsal bone, at the junction of the red and white skin.

Bladder-66: In the depression behind the fifth metatarsophalangeal joint.

INTERVENTIONS BY HEADACHE LOCATION

Rather than taking the wrong medication for a specific type of headache while you are experience a totally different kind, I'd like you to consider merely identifying the location on your head where the headache first began. Because pain travels and refers, it is important to focus on the origin of the pain, and also catch the headache at first sign of discomfort.

Simply find the corresponding head-image from the 4 illustrations below, and then take the appropriate steps to overcome the headache.

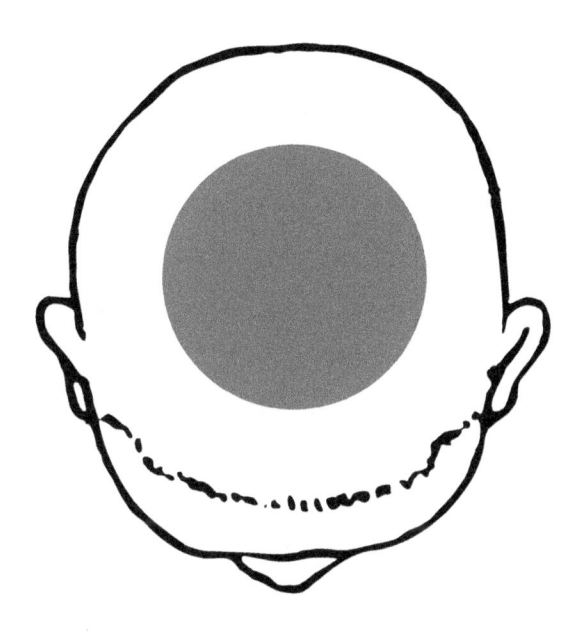

LOCATION #1:
Vertex - Top of the Head

When you feel a headache originate at the top of your head, it is most likely due to excessive toxins in the body and a stressed liver function.

Why it happens: The liver is responsible for purifying blood while the body is at rest and for maintaining the free-coursing of blood as needed for activities. When the liver is taxed due to excessive consumption of toxins (e.g., nitrates, mucus forming foods, pesticides, chemical medications, release of an abundance of stress hormones), it is unable to properly purify and move blood. The blood then circulates these toxins, and causes changes in body chemistry and blood vessel pressure. In addition, excessive alcohol consumption and prolonged angry emotions tend to further retard liver function, causing it to send energy upward as opposed to downward. With this, the face becomes flush, eyes turn red, and a headache erupts. Think anger headaches and hangovers.

What to do: There are several things that can be done to decrease a headache at this location depending on where you are and how much time you have:

- ✓ Drink two 8 oz. glasses of cool purified water.
- ✓ Immediately do 10 repetitions (slow and steady) of the two breathing exercises.
- ✓ Press, for 30 seconds each these two acu-points: Liver-2 and Liver-3
- ✓ Avoid all dairy, spicy, and nitrate-heavy foods.
- ✓ If you are able, administer yourself an enema to clear toxin-heavy stools from your bowels.

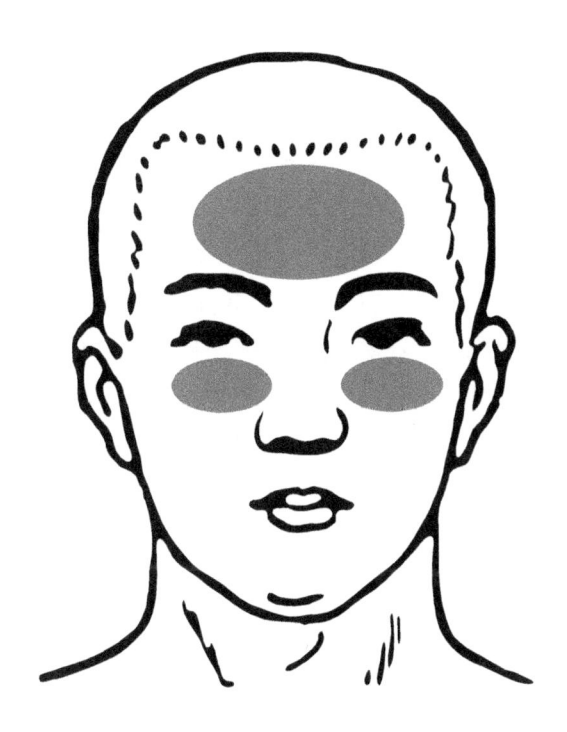

LOCATION #2:
The Face and Forehead

When you feel a headache originate on your face or forehead, it is generally caused by inflammation of the sinuses or excessive fat levels in the blood and lymph systems.

Why it happens: Inflammation of the face and forehead is generally caused by excessive dampness and mucus. Externally, this happens through changes in barometric pressure brought on by rain, snow or humidity. Internally, the dampness is caused by certain foods, like dairy, hydrogenated oils, and fats. This type of headache is related to the functions of the lung, stomach, large intestines, and gall bladder. This is why you feel sinus pressure and pain before a storm or after consuming too much dairy, fatty foods, and beverages.

What to do: There are several strategies available to prevent, reduce, and stop headaches that originate on the face or forehead.

- ✓ Drink strong ginger tea, no milk or sugar. Either cut up fresh ginger, add to boiling water and drink or buy ginger green or ginger white tea. No black or red tea.
- ✓ When eating on this day, add some ginger, scallion, and cayenne pepper to the dishes, as they promote sweating without causing further inflammation.
- ✓ Press for 30 seconds each, these two acu-points: Stomach-43 and 44.
- ✓ Avoid ALL dairy products the day the headache presents and the following day.
- ✓ Avoid all fats and oils the day the headache presents and the following day.
- ✓ If your environment is damp or musty, use a dehumidifier and turn up the heat to dry it out.

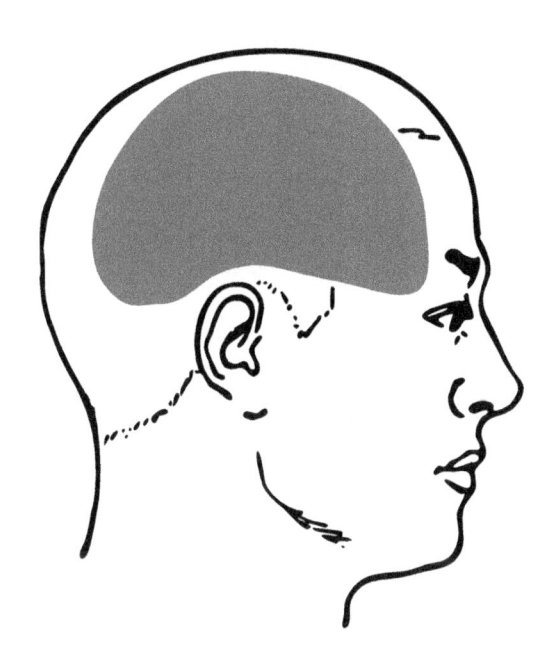

LOCATION #3:
Temples and Behind the Eyes

Headaches occurring at the temples, behind the eyes or like a band around the head at the templar area are related to stressed function of the gallbladder, kidneys, lungs, and liver. These headaches tend to be a combination of the above two due to impure blood, lymph, toxins, and dampness merging all at once to cause pain that often leads to sweating, shaking, and vomiting.

Why it happens: Pressure and pain occur around the temples, behind the eyes, and around the head as a reaction against excessive dampness and toxins in the lymph and blood systems. Through weather patterns, physical live/work location or dietary choices, accumulation of toxins and mucus forms in the body and obstructs the vessels and channels, causing pressure and pain.

What to do: Since templar and eye headaches are a combination of the previously described headaches, you can prevent them by following those steps. Given the potential severity of this headache, it is best to do everything mentioned as soon as headache onset is felt (or assumed to be coming).

- ✓ Drink ginger tea, and cook with ginger, scallions, and cayenne pepper to induce sweating and expel toxins.
- ✓ Drink two 8 oz. glasses of purified water to hydrate and flush the kidneys.
- ✓ Immediately do 10 repetitions of the "Toxin-Reducing Breathing" exercise.
- ✓ Press these two acu-points for 30 seconds each: Gallbladder-34 and 43.
- ✓ Avoid ALL of the following foods: Milk, cheese, yogurt, ice cream, hydrogenated and partially-hydrogenated oils, fatty meats, refined white sugar, caffeine (coffee, black tea, soda), artificial sweeteners, and nitrates (cold cuts, hot dogs, cured meats).

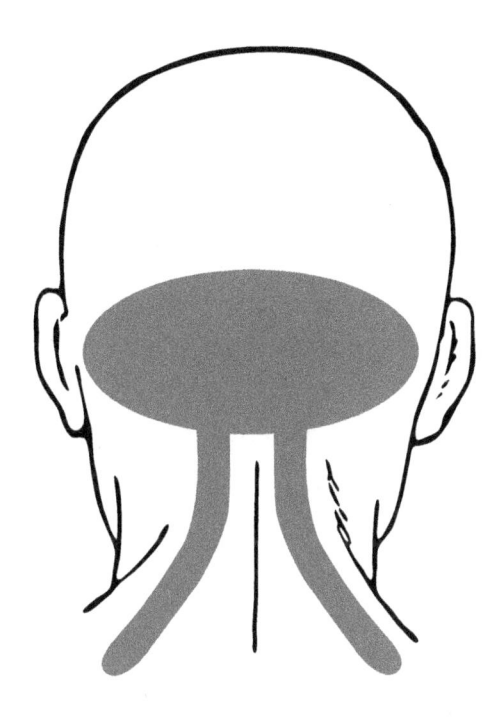

LOCATION #4:
Occiput – Base of the Skull

Headaches originating at the back of the head are generally cause by muscle contraction or irritation of the trigeminal nerve. They can be triggered by stress, improper posture, excessive exercise, and toxins affecting the function of the kidneys, bladder, and liver.

Why it happens: Physical tension is the main culprit behind occipital headaches or those that start at the base of the skull or upper cervical neck regions. By sitting with poor posture, lifting heavy objects or engaging in an activity where the arms are held above the head for a prolonged periods of time, the muscles of the shoulders, neck and occipital region of the head spasm in their natural attempt at holding the body erect. Emotional and psychological stress can also lead to cramping of these muscles and headaches to the back of the head. The muscle contractions either compress spinal vertebrae or irritate cervical nerves and cause pain that refers up and around from the back of the head toward the front.

What to do: The easiest way to prevent an occipital headache is to prevent the muscles of the shoulders, neck, and base of the skull from contracting. Here are things to do to prevent this, and also relax them when they do tense.

- ✓ Drink two 8 oz. glasses of cool, purified water.
- ✓ At onset of tightness or pain in the shoulders, neck or base of the skull, take a break from what you are doing and perform 3 to 6 very slow sets of the "Shoulder and Neck Stretches."
- ✓ Press these two acu-points for 30 seconds each: Bladder-65 and 66.
- ✓ Immediately correct and always maintain proper seated and sleeping postures to prevent spinal misalignment and muscle spasm trigger points.
- ✓ Reduce daily stress by performing the two breathing exercises before drifting off to sleep, and, as often as needed, to reduce stress by balancing respiration.

CHAPTER REVIEW

- With so many headache types and symptoms, finding the right intervention or medication for them can be difficult. It is especially difficult when chronic sufferers tend to experience more than one headache type at a time.

- An easier solution is to feel the headache and identify which part(s) of the head is affected. Then use the intervention specific to that (those) area(s) at the *first sign* of a headache.

- I urge you to copy these interventions and keep them in your coat pocket, desk, at work, bag or anyplace else so they are handy at all times. When you start to feel a headache, use these techniques first before taking medication! (We are trying to break a pain-meds-pain loop).

- In all cases, while integrating "The Headache Relief Action Plan" into your new lifestyle, attempt to only use medication when you absolutely need it. First, change your diet, sleep, etc as outlined and then utilize the intervention for relief, and only when that fails, go for the meds.

- The more elements of the program you can embrace, the less and less you will need any pain-killing pill.

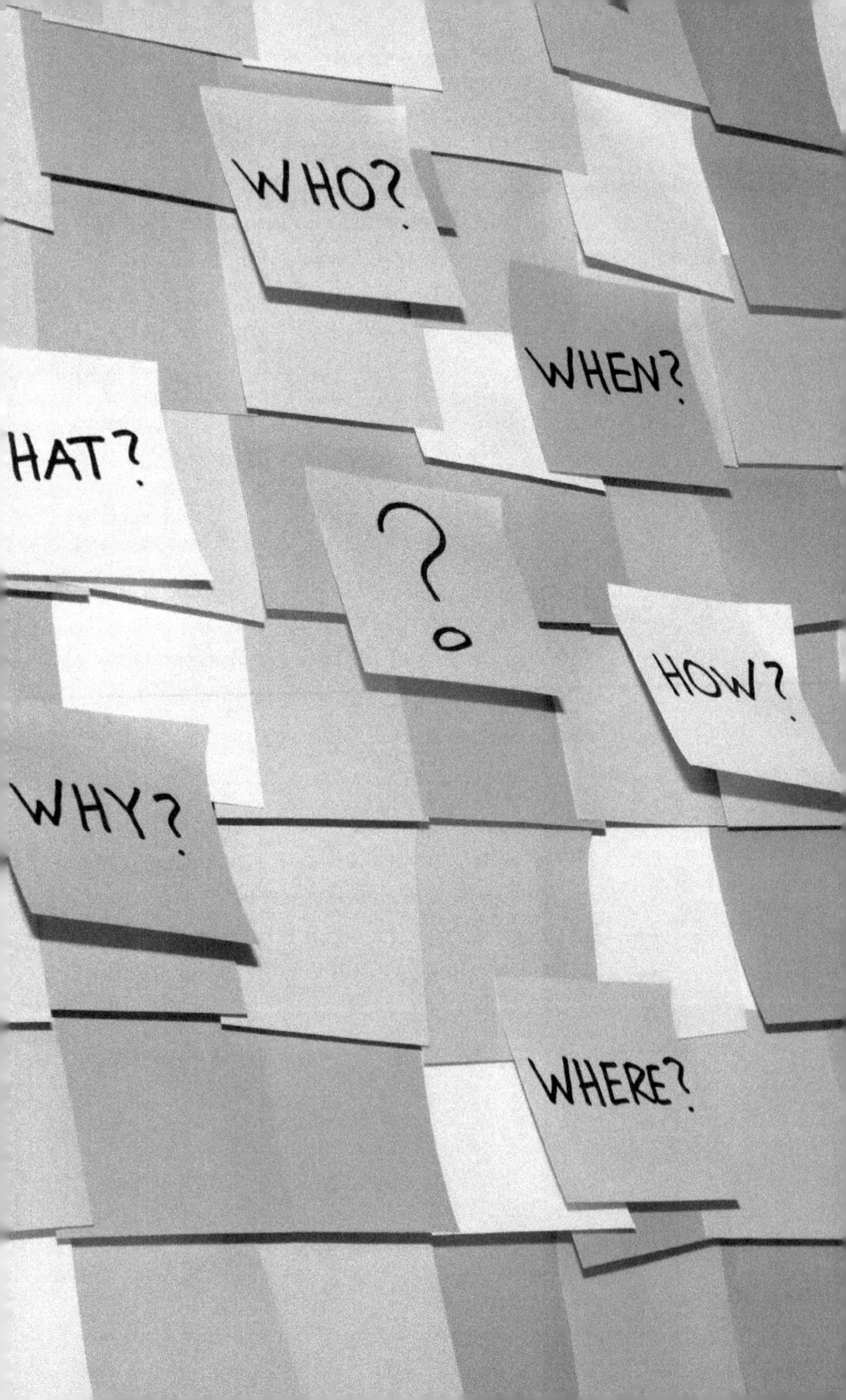
WHO?
WHEN?
HAT?
?
HOW?
WHY?
WHERE?

PART 3

THE 30-DAY HEADACHE RELIEF ACTION PLAN

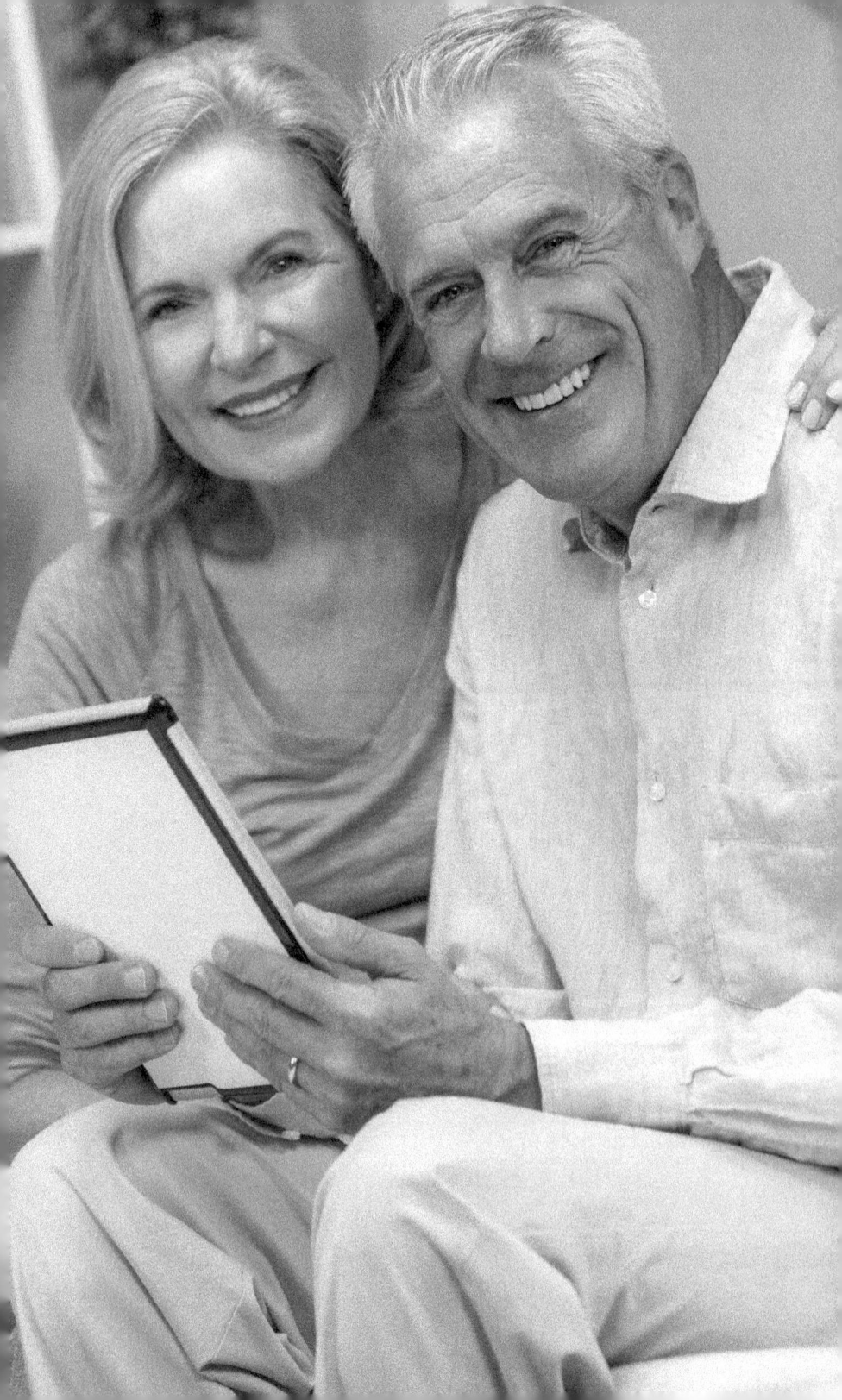

CHAPTER 20

INTRODUCTION TO THE HEADACHE RELIEF ACTION PLAN

For many headache sufferers, headaches seem to be an inevitable part of life. In fact, you can take preventive measures to reduce your pain or completely escape it. But first, you have to recognize what is bringing on those debilitating aches.

In fact, hundreds of thousands of headaches pound inside the heads of people every day. As mentioned previously, most of these episodes are completely preventable and are caused by the choices each headache sufferer makes. Yes, I am saying that we create, cause, and trigger our own headaches. And because of that simple truth, you can stop doing what you are doing and prevent your headaches from ever coming back. That's a fact I want you to fully embrace as you embark on the path to a headache-free life by implementing "The Headache Relief Action Plan."

So why are there still so many chapters before "The Headache Relief Action Plan" is outlined? Simply because knowing the types of headaches (presented in Part 1) and knowing the solutions to overcoming headache triggers (outlined in Part 2) don't seem to be enough for success. There is a third part, which is how to be successful with this program in areas where others may have failed.

Accountability — Headaches do not just appear out of thin air. We'd like to think they do because no one wants to be held accountable for their own pain. People who suffer chronic headaches (and I was one of them for more than 30 years), often feel like powerless victims who are dependent on drugs and various therapies to lessen the suffering.

Rethink the situation this way: You can be considered cured of chronic headaches if you successfully *prevent* them from occurring. The cure is in the prevention, not in a response to the symptoms or in a therapy to reduce the symptoms. No amount of drugs or other therapies can ever cure your headaches because these measures are not designed to stop them from occurring.

And so to be successful you must be accountable to yourself for aligning with the program strategies and methods, which require lifestyle and attitude changes. You can do it and this section walks you through the steps of what to do to be successful in the program. These steps include:

A Positive Attitude Supports a Successful Program — Healthy people are happy people; and shifting your attitude from "nothing helps" to "I can make better choices" is often the key step that offers optimal wellness and emotional fulfillment. Health and happiness represent a frame of mind that influences your choices. In turn, making better lifestyle choices leads to wellness instead of chronic ill health. "The Headache Relief Action Plan" is grounded in headache relief and prevention methods; however, without a positive attitude from the start, success will be difficult.

Setting SMART Goals — Reaching your headache and migraine relief goals can be a difficult task. For many people, tackling such tasks, let alone setting goals to do so, can be daunting. But I want you to know that you can achieve your headache relief and prevention goals by implementing a simple tool to help you develop and stay on track. The tool is a goal-setting concept called SMART. Each letter stands for the word that represents a component of an effective plan: **S**pecific, **M**easurable, **A**ttainable, **R**ealistic, and **T**imely.

Program Objectives and Strategies — The power of "The Headache Relief Action Plan" is based on its structure. I cannot stress enough that for best results with this program, you must understand the headache and migraine process, the components involved in reducing the triggers, frequency, level and duration of headaches, and how to create a positive attitude and set SMART goals to create an environment for success. Without all of this in place, it may be difficult to believe in the program, fully commit to doing it and seeing it through. If you've read everything from my personal message through Chapter 19, then you're well on your way to achieving program success and lasting relief from chronic headaches and migraines.

Getting Started: The First Three Days — One of the main reasons people claim they have started and stopped diet plans and workout routines is because they could not "get into" the program fully due to the first three days being overwhelming for them. I have also crashed and burned within the first three days of my own health goals over the years, but was lucky to find a solution to this problem.

Step-by-Step: The 30-Day Headache Relief Action Plan — Now it's time to put into harmonious action the hundreds of pieces of information from this book into a wellness lifestyle that supports relief from headaches and migraines and reversal of its symptoms. Below are charts outlining the seven major categories discussed in this book, and the solutions associated with each. Implementing solutions from each of these categories forms the essence of "The Headache Relief Action Plan." The charts give you guidance into selecting best options within each category. You must, however, review the individual chapters to find the specific details of each solution and consider which ones resonate best with you.

I cannot stress enough the importance of reading all these chapters. Also, while adopting the program as part of your new lifestyle, you'll continue to get headaches (just fewer and less painful over time). When these occur, and when you feel their "first sign" of coming on, please do not reach for medication; instead, utilize the specific pain location interventions I presented in Chapter 19. If they don't work for you, take the minimum of meds you can to get by and continue on with the program. With each passing week, you will see greater and greater improvements in how you feel and a reduction in headache days, intensity, and the duration of headaches.

Good luck!

CHAPTER 21

A POSITIVE ATTITUDE SUPPORTS A SUCCESSFUL PROGRAM

If you want to be healthy and happy instead of pained and sick, it may be necessary to readjust your attitude toward health. I know what you're thinking, "I didn't choose to be a headache sufferer. It's not my choice to be in chronic pain and not be able to fully live my life. I see specialists and practitioners to help my condition." I hear you. I know you are making your way forward in the best way you know how.

HEALTHY THOUGHT PROCESSES

Studies show that healthy people seem to share certain characteristics. In fact, these characteristics are so prevalent among the healthy that those who share them could be considered a demographic. We are all familiar with demographics constructed around ethnicity, age, gender, and income. But did you know there is a demographic of the population that is concerned with a healthy lifestyle and green technology?

There is, and it's called LOHAS (Lifestyles of Health and Sustainability). LOHAS.com defines the group as, "A market segment focused on health and fitness, the environment, personal development, sustainable living, and social justice."

Not everyone who qualifies as part of the LOHAS demographic gains entrance by virtue of being healthy, pain-free, and happy. However, it does seem that once people embrace this lifestyle, they become healthier and happier. Why? Because they have shifted their mindset, their perspective, from one of "nothing helps" and "I have to live with my pain" to "there are choices I can make to better myself."

Do you need to embrace LOHAS to be healthy and happy? No. Maybe worrying about green technology, carbon footprints, renewable resources, and social justice is not your thing. But being healthy, pain-free, free of chronic illness, and living a vibrant and fulfilling life is something I think most people want.

I would like to share with you the characteristics (e.g., thoughts, actions and behaviors) most common among those who are healthy. And if you recall from several previous chapters of this book, what we think, do, and feel all contribute to headache cause and prevention. If you can begin embracing the below outlined healthy thoughts, actions, and behaviors (even one at a time), you should see improvement, not only in your chronic headaches but also in your health overall as well as significant improvement in your quality of life.

BELIEVE YOU CAN IMPROVE YOUR WELLNESS

While you may never be cured of your current health conditions, you can make vast progress in a short amount of time by having a better mindset and making better choices. A belief that your condition can improve is the motivational force necessary to begin feeling better. One small change at a time leads to many broader changes over time, which can then make dramatic shifts in your headache frequency, duration, and pain.

OWN YOUR PRESENT STATE OF HEALTH

Whether you see a medical doctor or alternative health practitioner, leaving your health in their hands may not significantly improve your condition. Owning your condition, taking responsibility for it, and doing what you need to do to improve yourself are characteristics of healthy people. When you're mildly sick, do what you need to do to get well to prevent yourself from becoming seriously ill. Your health is yours, and no one cares as much as you do about improving it. Healthy people know this and take steps to promote wellness, not hinder it.

KNOW YOU CAN DO IT YOURSELF…
WITH A LITTLE HELP

Roughly 80% of all conditions of pain, illness, and disease are self-induced. That is to say, they are caused by the person who is suffering from them. The problem is two-fold: people don't know their condition is self-induced and they don't know what they are doing to cause it. As a result, they don't know what to do to change it. Healthy people acknowledge they cause their illness and then change course from their usual choices and behaviors, knowing they can choose better and prevent them.

MAKE CHOICES AND STICK TO THEM

One of the most difficult things people grapple with is sticking with a program for change. We choose to join the gym, but don't go. We make a series of appointments with the acupuncturist, but attend only three out of 10. Making strong wellness choices puts you on the path to wellness. Sticking with them and seeing them through keeps you on the wellness path. Healthy people make healthy choices and stick with those choices, even when they are tired, under the weather or busy. And this characteristic is intertwined with the other three: belief, ownership, and knowledge.

KEEP AN OPEN MIND

Health and wellness solutions come in all shapes and sizes. A few decades ago, chiropractic medicine was seen as quackery, but today it is a mainstream therapy. Ten years ago, acupuncture was still foreign to most Americans. While energy healing, meditation, polarity therapy, Reiki, and herbal therapy may seem strange to you and part of the fringe, healthy people keep an open mind about what can improve their wellness. They may not understand something, but their exploratory nature and drive for a wellness lifestyle allow them to look into it, ask questions, interview a practitioner, and experience an introductory session or class. Just because you are unfamiliar with a healing concept does not mean the solution is quackery. Keeping an open mind to new ideas and solutions can lead to an improved state of wellness.

MAKE WELLNESS A LIFESTYLE

The most important aspect of wellness is the fact that healthy people on the whole tend to make wellness a focal point of their lifestyle. If you carry a perspective of wellness with you when grocery shopping, you choose ingredients and foods that promote wellness, such as organic fruits and vegetables. When thinking of an afternoon activity during lunch break, the wellness-minded person may choose a walk or quiet time rather than kvetching in the break room about co-workers that bother them. Rather than watching TV for two hours after dinner, the wellness lifestyle may find you doing yoga, stretching or meditating instead.

If your goal is to stop suffering by improving your overall health condition, then living a wellness lifestyle is a means to this end. There is an entire demographic of healthy and happy people doing it. You can do it, too. Do you need to fully embrace the LOHAS lifestyle and join the demographic to become well? No. But I'll bet that over time your wellness choices will impact your well-being and you will want to.

CHAPTER REVIEW

- Health and happiness can overcome pain and sickness when you readjust your attitude toward a healthy frame of mind that influences your choices.
- By making better lifestyle choices, you can find wellness instead of chronic ill health.
- Model the thoughts, actions, and behaviors of those who are healthy and happy.
- Believe you can improve your wellness and prevent your headaches.
- Own your present state of health so you can actively change it.
- Know you can do it yourself, but will require a little help from others.
- Make good choices and stick with them.
- Make wellness a part of your lifestyle!

CHAPTER 22

SETTING SMART WELLNESS GOALS FOR SUCCESS

Reaching your headache and migraine relief goals — or any wellness goal for that matter — can be a difficult task. For many people, tackling such tasks, let alone setting goals to do so, can be daunting. Often times the perceived effort it will take to undertake the activities to achieve the goals, and the time involved, seems more difficult than remaining in place. Thus, many people fall short of achieving their wellness goals or end up doing nothing to achieve them.

I know you have been suffering for a long time, and that you have tried many therapies. But I want you to know that you can achieve your headache relief and prevention goals by implementing a simple tool to help you develop and stay on track. The tool is a goal-setting concept called SMART. Each letter stands for the word that represents a component of an effective plan:

Specific
Measurable
Attainable
Realistic
Timely

Each of these five components is essential to both creating and achieving your wellness goals. Let's look at them individually in more detail.

SPECIFIC

The more specific you can make your goals, the better the chance you have of achieving them. Specificity allows for understanding and measuring success along the other four areas of SMART. Without specificity, you will do more floating on the ocean than sailing on the seas. Driving in circles is never as fun or satisfying as directly reaching your destination. The more specific the details of the trip, the sooner you can reach the destination. And there can be more than one destination – a series of mini destinations – on the way to reaching the big destination over time. When working toward specificity, it is a good idea to begin by considering the five Ws: Why, What, Who, Where, and When.

Why you want to change your state of health is the most important decision you can verbalize because it fuels your desire and sets your level of commitment to the program overall. Without knowing why, it is easy to do nothing.

What you want to accomplish is the next decision. Do you want to improve your diet or reduce the frequency of your headaches? The *what* of the matter is important for deciding on…

Who you need to involve. Wellness programs work best with a support structure in place. Who will you involve in the achievement of your goals? How about a workout neighbor, massage therapist, moral support from a loved one or a health care provider? Once these are all in place you will know...

Where all of this needs to happen. Do you require visits to an acupuncturist or just a quiet place to meditate each day? What about the local yoga class or your living room?

When all this comes into play, it is important for setting schedules and staying on track. People do better and reach their goals faster when they are in a routine. Knowing when to do what you need is important to establish before you begin. Being specific is essential to knowing what goals you want to achieve and how to get there.

MEASURABLE

Having measurable goals and a reliable metrics system are essential for achieving wellness goals. After all, without measuring progress, how will you know if you've reached your goal or mini-stops along the way? There are two parts to "measurable;" the measured goal and the criteria for measuring it.

Let's say your goal is to lose 20 pounds in six months. Standing on a scale once per week offers the metric. Making a chart of progress at the end of each month, and measuring that against your hoped-for mini-monthly goals gives you the criteria for measurement. Other scales are also available: A 1-10 subjective scales for things like pain; hour scales for time (important for sleep measurements); or pH readings for your body's acidity level and so on.

The first step is to create a list of what you want to measure, and then how it can be measured. How much weight do you want to lose? How many minutes of meditation or sessions of stretching do you want to do each week? How much of a decrease in pain do you want to feel each week, each month, over what time? Being "specific" about these "measurements" will help you decide what is "attainable." These measuring tools are provided as part of "The Headache Relief Action Plan."

ATTAINABLE

There is a truism that advises, "If you can imagine it, you can achieve it." I have put this to the test many times and succeeded, and so can you! But the achieving is more likely to be attainable if the goals and vision are realistic enough to actually be attained. You must set an objective that you personally feel is obtainable and for which you are willing to put forth the effort. You can desire a long-off goal, but setting markers of achievement along the way will make it more attainable.

Many quit their wellness routines or drop their wellness lifestyles when they do not attain their desired goals in an immediate time frame because they lack honest "mile markers." Listing small goals that will lead to larger goals is not only a successful way of attaining measurable results, but of building your self-confidence, self-belief, and self-image.

REALISTIC

In order for wellness goals to be attainable and measurable, they must be realistic for you. That is, they need to be something you are physically, mentally, and financially able to achieve. What identifies as realistic is a matter of personal relevance; you are the only one who can distinguish this.

Returning to an earlier example, if it's your goal to lose 20 pounds, this must be realistic for you. If you are sufficiently overweight, then losing 20 pounds makes healthy sense. But if you are not, then losing this much weight may be unrealistic and also unhealthy. Do you have the time and dedication to work toward achieving that goal? Do you have the financial and structural support necessary to allow it to happen? Moreover, being realistic means giving yourself several months to lose the weight, and not just a few weeks. Setting realistic time frames will go a long way to keeping you on track.

TIMELY

Timeliness is an important part of goal setting, especially when it comes to wellness. In what time frame are you hoping to achieve your goals? How much time per day, week, and month are you planning on dedicating to the attainment of those goals? What time of day are you able to do this, and fit it in with your overall life schedule? Being specific regarding your time is crucial. Just saying that you are "working on getting healthy" or on "the path of headache prevention" is a statement that can lead to failure. Timeframes are important for goals to be measured in a meaningful, realistic, and attainable way. You must be specific. And to help you with this, "The Headache Relief Action Plan" is structured into 30-day plans.

Once you have spent some time considering all of this and listing out the specifics of each of the five components, it's time to write out your SMART action statement. Here is an example to help you come up with your own:

> *"I want to feel better and experience less pain because it makes me feel good, and when I feel good, I enjoy my life. I will lose 20 pounds and decrease my pain by 50%. To do this I will need the support of my family, a dietician and a personal trainer, who is available on Wednesdays and Sundays. I will use a scale and a pain index to chart my*

progress over the next six months with mini goals set at the end of each month. I believe I can attain my goal because the time frame is realistic. I have a support system. I know what I need to do. I believe in myself and I am dedicated to changing my own life for the better."

This statement is generic, but speaks to each of the five components of the SMART wellness goal-setting concept. Try it and see what a difference it can make in reaching your personal fitness, health and wellness goals. Let's now move on and discuss, specifically, the goals, objectives and strategies of the Headache Relief Action Plan.

CHAPTER REVIEW

- Use the goal-setting concept called SMART to reach your headache relief goals.
- Specific goals create better chances of actualizing them.
- Measurable goals combined with reliable metrics are essential.
- Attainable goals must also be realistic enough to be achieved.
- Timeliness is critical in setting goals for success.
- The success of your "Headache Relief Action Plan" must be combined with SMART goals.

CHAPTER 23

PROGRAM STRATEGIES, OBJECTIVES AND METRICS

Here you are at Chapter 23, where you finally get to read an overview of "The Headache Relief Action Plan." If you've read the book from the beginning, you will have a much better and more global understanding of headaches and migraines. If you have not read the book from the beginning, please stop and do so. I cannot stress enough that for best results with this program, you must understand the headache and migraine process, the components involved in reducing triggers, frequency, level, and duration of headaches, and how to create a positive attitude and set SMART goals to create an environment for success.

Without all of this in place, it may be difficult to believe in the program, fully commit to doing it, and seeing it through. If you have read everything from my personal message through Chapter 22, then you're well on your way to achieving program success and lasting relief from chronic headaches and migraines.

The power of "The Headache Relief Action Plan" is based on its structure. I developed it with an integrated Mind-Body-Diet approach for a strong through-line (or scaffold) on which the various program segments are hung. We could also look at it like a tree: The roots are the information and knowledge upon which the program (tree) grows; the tree is the structure on which the program is based; and the branches are the actions and methods that will create positive change.

"The Headache Relief Action Plan" is based on the following five "structures:"

1. Gaining knowledge of headaches
2. Having a strategy for success
3. Creating a personal vision statement
4. Setting long-term goals
5. Establishing short-term objectives

If you have read the book from the beginning, then the first structure – gaining information-based knowledge – is already complete. Let's now take a look at our strategy for optimizing the success of "The Headache Relief Action Plan."

THE STRATEGY FOR SUCCESS

Without a strategy, not much can be accomplished. The most successful generals were victorious in battle partly because they had a successful strategy. Well, those who are at war with a debilitating, chronic headache or migraine condition need a strategy to overcome it. The strategy I developed for you is based on these principles:

1. Taking a DIY (Do-It-Yourself) approach is the only way to fully embrace the program, create wellness goals,

Program Strategies, Objectives and Metrics

change your environment, alter your lifestyle choices to healthier options, and create a better quality of life.

2. Seeking outside help as needed for specific things, including various hands-on therapies like bodywork, massage, FMS and BAUD therapy, acupuncture, fitness instruction, and assisted stretching.

3. Using the SMART concept to help achieve success, by being realistic about expectations and getting friends, family, and co-workers onboard for support.

4. Embracing a natural and integrated mind-body- diet approach to change all aspects of your life needed to achieve positive results that last.

5. Creating personal long-term goals, and short-term objectives by using various metrics to establish your current "set point" and track your progress moving forward.

6. Having everything ready to go before beginning the program. Use the four days prior to the "first three days" to swap out bad foods and drinks for good ones. Have your first round of supplements and pain-relieving topical products on hand, and have appointments set for consultations or actual appointments with three wellness practitioners.

7. Being focused and ready to roll on day one because you've read this book, have the knowledge of the situation, belief in the program, and an "I am motivated!" attitude.

Now that you can see there are well thought-out strategies in place, you should be more confident in the program and your ability to be successful in it. Let's turn that strategy into something more tangible by fleshing out its pieces as they relate to you personally.

CREATE YOUR PERSONAL VISION STATEMENT

Creating your own personal Vision Statement is a great way to set a view of what you want to do and who you wish to become. How do you envision yourself now, the process of change, and where you will be on the other end? To help you get started, here is my personal Vision Statement:

> *"My vision is to widen the reach of holistic wellness, bringing its message and methods to a broader audience through books, articles, webinars, personal health coaching, and corporate wellness consulting."*

Here is an example of a Vision Statement a person with headaches and migraines going through my program might write:

> *"My vision is to become self-empowered, to take personal control of my thoughts, emotions and actions to fully embrace Dr. Wiley's self-directed headache program so I may reduce my pain, increase my range of motion, change my life in positive ways that support wellness, and to finally regain control of my life and be happy."*

Think about it for a moment and then try writing a statement of your own. Do this on a separate piece of paper or on your computer. When you have a succinct and empowering personal Vision Statement, write it below. You will refer back to this as you progress in the program.

My personal vision is to... _____

_____

_____

SET YOUR LONG-TERM GOALS

Goal-setting is another powerful way to align yourself with your vision and the outcomes you desire. Without goals (general long-term desires) and objectives (specific short-term expectations), we lack the focus necessary to move forward in positive and productive ways.

You can have more than one goal as long as they generically speak to the achievement or accomplishment of aspects of the program or your health and are based on implementing the methods outlined in this book.

Goals are defined as *the purpose toward which an endeavor is directed, and the results achieved from them.* Here are examples of a few generic goals someone suffering chronic headaches might have:

Personal Goal - Example 1: My goal is to decrease the number of headaches I get each month, the numbers of days I am affected by those headaches, and the level of pain of each so I can feel better and enjoy a better quality of life.

Personal Goal - Example 2: My goal is to reduce my stress, improve my sleep, release held tensions in my body, and prevent my headache triggers in order to improve my quality of life.

Please take some time to write down several of your own goals on a separate piece of paper. Once you have them as you like, write them down in the space provided below. You will refer back to them as you go through the program.

Goal #1: _____

_____

_____

_____

_____

_____

_____

Goal #2: _____

_____

_____

_____

_____

Program Strategies, Objectives and Metrics

Goal #3: _____

_____

_____

_____

_____

_____

_____

ESTABLISH YOUR SHORT-TERM OBJECTIVES

Objectives are the specific targets you want to reach within the larger goal you set for yourself. Unlike goals, objectives are set for the short-term and are matched to metrics. In the case of our headache program, those metrics include pain, frequency and duration, diet, stress, tightness in shoulders and neck, sleep quality, and more.

Personal Objective – Example 1: I aim to embrace the headache-prevention diet plan and add supplementation to it within the first week to help kick-start my success in "The Headache Relief Action Plan."

Personal Objective – Example 2: I aim to see a massage therapist, BAUD therapist, and a personal trainer within the first month and attend all the required sessions.

Personal Objective – Example 3: I will follow the guidelines provided to change my sleeping environment and posture and get an average of eight hours of reparative sleep every night by the first week of the program.

Please take some time to write down several of your own objectives on a separate piece of paper. Once you have them as you like, write them down in the space provided below. You will refer back to them as you go through the program.

Objective #1: _____

_____

_____

_____

_____

_____

_____

Objective #2: _____

_____

_____

_____

_____

_____

_____

Program Strategies, Objectives and Metrics

Objective #3: _____

_____
_____
_____
_____
_____
_____
_____

Objective #4: _____

_____
_____
_____
_____
_____
_____
_____

Objective #5: _____

_____
_____
_____
_____
_____
_____
_____

USE METRICS TO ASSESS YOUR "SET-POINT"

Metrics are an important aspect of any program that has a certain success level as its goal. To reduce and then prevent chronic headaches and migraines, metrics are essential. They objectively quantify certain parts of the program and subjectively qualify how you are feeling along the way. I can't tell you how many times I treated patients for mixed pain syndrome (different kinds of pain in various places in the body), and then had them tell me they don't feel any different. I would then take out the patient metrics chart, which was subjectively filled in by the patient, and show them that their headaches are down 45%, their sleep has improved by 60%, and their inflammation is down by 70%. And, of course, they would say, "Yes, but my elbow still hurts!"

I joke; but in all seriousness, you need a subjective assessment of several things to effectively implement "The Headache Relief Action Plan" and be successful. Like your Vision Statement, goals, and objectives, your personal metrics need to be written down. However, these also need to be updated every week as long as you are on the program. This way, you will be able to chart everything each week and compare it with previous weeks on the program and with how you felt before beginning the program. This will let you know how you are doing in each of the essential aspects of what it takes to reduce the frequency, pain, and duration of your chronic headaches and then prevent them from occurring again. Here are the areas to apply metrics to, and what you need to do.

Metric 1: Pain. Using Mosby's "Pain Rating Scale," please circle the number that most closely reflects how much pain you feel on a daily basis.

Program Strategies, Objectives and Metrics

Pain Rating Scale ©Mosby

No Pain   Worst Possible Pain

0   1   2   3   4   5   6   7   8   9   10
None   Mild   Moderate   Severe

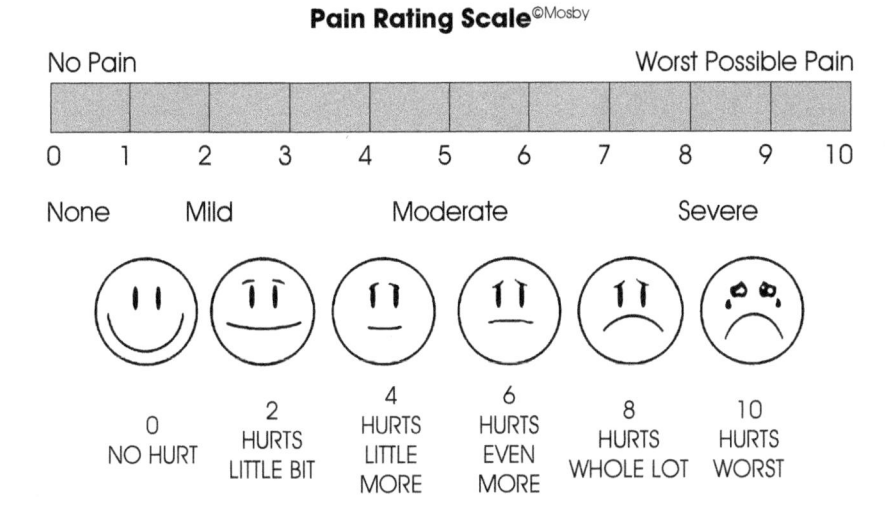

0	2	4	6	8	10
NO HURT	HURTS LITTLE BIT	HURTS LITTLE MORE	HURTS EVEN MORE	HURTS WHOLE LOT	HURTS WORST

Metric 2. Emotional State. Using the "Emotions Scale," please consider your overall feelings about yourself in relation to your headaches. You can circle all the feelings you experience on a daily basis related to headaches and migraines, but please only select one number for your baseline rating.

Low   Neutral   High

0   1   2   3   4   5   6   7   8   9   10

panic	angry	bored	playful	happy	excited
helpless	sad	fed up	content	satisfied	joyful
rage	scared	annoyed			ecstatic
apathetic	disappointed				
grieving	upset				

Metric 3 – Stress: Measuring stress can be tricky because so many things are involved. There is both good and bad stress, and what is more important is how well one deals with their daily stress. If you are interested in taking a comprehensive stress test, I recommend visiting www.freestresstest.org and take their 100-question, online test. For our purposes, please rate your stress level based on this question:

Thinking about the last month, how stressed do you subjectively feel when compared to times when you felt "life was good?"

Stress Feeling	Level
Not At All Stressed	0
Seldom Stressed	1-2
Sometimes Stressed	3-4
Frequently Stressed	5-6
Chronically Stressed	7-8
Nervous Breakdown*	9-10

*If you are feeling you may be on the verge of a nervous breakdown, please seek immediate medical attention or call a local therapist for help.

Metric 4 – Sleep Quality: Getting good quality sleep is essential to feeling better since this is when the body repairs itself. Good quality sleep means sleeping in the correct posture for seven to eight hours per night, seven days per week, without disturbance, and awaking feeling refreshed. Given these qualifications, how would you rate your quality of sleep overall, over the past month? Circle one answer for each of the three qualifications, and then add your answers to get your total sleep quality score.

Sleep Quality	Poor = 1	Good = 2	Great = 3
Sleep Position	Stomach	Back	Side
Sleep Hours	4-6 hrs	6.5 7 hrs	7.5-8 hrs
Awaking Refreshed	Never	Sometimes	Always
Total Score = ___			

Metric 5 – Body Mass Index (BMI): The Body Mass Index (BMI) measures your height to weight ratio. A BMI between 18.5-24.9 is within a healthy limit. Above or below is not so healthy. Please find the BMI number that connects your height and weight in the below "Body Mass Index Calculator."

BMI Chart

Height \ Weight [pounds]	100	110	120	130	140	150	160	170	180	190	200	210	220	230	240	250	260
4'6"	24	27	29	31	34	36	39	41	43	46	48	51	53	55	58	60	63
4'8"	22	25	27	29	31	34	36	38	40	43	45	47	49	52	54	56	58
4'10"	21	23	25	27	29	31	33	36	38	40	42	44	46	48	50	52	54
5'0"	20	21	23	25	27	29	31	33	35	37	39	41	43	45	47	49	51
5'2"	18	20	22	24	26	27	29	31	33	35	37	38	40	42	44	46	48
5'4"	17	19	21	22	24	26	27	29	31	33	34	36	38	39	41	43	45
5'6"	16	18	19	21	23	24	26	27	29	31	32	34	36	37	39	40	42
5'8"	15	17	18	20	21	23	24	26	27	29	30	32	33	35	36	38	40
5'10"	14	16	17	19	20	22	23	24	26	27	29	30	32	33	34	36	37
6'0"	14	15	16	18	19	20	22	23	24	26	27	28	30	31	33	34	35
6'2"	13	14	15	17	18	19	21	22	23	24	26	27	28	30	31	32	33
6'4"	12	13	15	16	17	18	19	21	22	23	24	26	27	28	29	30	32
6'6"	12	13	14	15	16	17	18	20	21	22	23	24	25	27	28	29	30
6'8"	11	12	13	14	15	16	18	19	20	21	22	23	24	25	26	27	29
6'10"	10	12	13	14	15	16	17	18	19	20	21	22	23	24	25	26	27
7'0"	10	11	12	13	14	15	16	17	18	19	20	21	22	23	24	25	26

Underweight | Normal Range | Overweight | Obese

Metric 6 – pH Level: pH is a measure of the acid to alkaline level in your body. A pH of seven is neutral, and above eight is alkaline (healthy). The lower the number, the more acidic (unhealthy) your body is. Please go to your local convenience store or pharmacy and purchase a set of pH testing strips (they are inexpensive). You will use either your saliva or urine to get a reading. Then circle your number on the chart below.

ACIDIC   ALKALINE

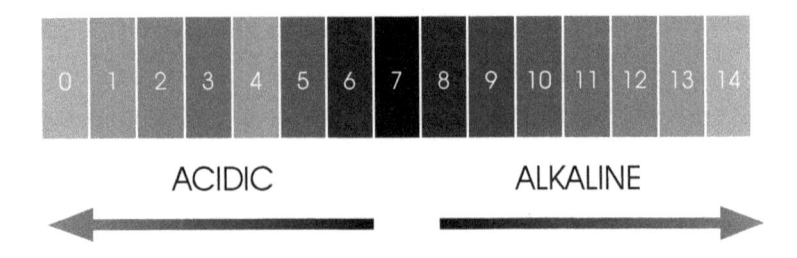

Metric 7 – Physical Activity: One of the worst things that people suffering from headaches deal with is their inability to do physical activity as they once did. But as you've learned, keeping active and moving the body is essential to preventing headaches and being healthy. Thinking back on the past month when compared to your "healthy prime," how subjectively do you feel you are able to exercise, walk, and do physical activities?

- I continue to exercise and do things as if I never had headaches = 1 - 2
- I have lost the ability to do some of the physical activities I enjoy = 3 - 4 - 5
- Headaches restrict many of the physical activities I used to do = 6 - 7- 8
- Headaches have made it nearly impossible to do any physical activity = 9 - 10

YOUR HEADACHES METRICS CHART

Please fill in the below chart with your "Set-Point" metrics from the above lines. Together, these numbers will give you a snapshot of your condition and tell you how you feel now, prior to beginning the program. Then, after beginning the program and at the time allocated on the chart, please re-do your metrics and enter your new numbers into the chart. It would be great if you see steady progress over the course of a few weeks to a few months.

However, it is not uncommon to feel a bit worse off at first, at least in some of the areas. This occurs because the body is being moved off its set point and led back toward balance (homeostasis). However, since suffering chronic headaches or even before then, it has found its new groove (a false sense of "balance") from being stuck in a symptomatic negative holding pattern.

Your Headache Metrics							
Pain Level	Set Point	7 Days	14 Days	21 Days	30 Days	60 Days	90 Days
Emotional State							
Stress Level							
Sleep Quality							
Body Mass Index							
pH Measure							
Range of Motion							
Physical Activity							

Please know that while it is easy to think that having "bad scores" means there is no hope for you, in actuality the opposite is true. *Those headache sufferers with the Highest Set Point have the greatest room for improvement* and therefore have *the best chance for marked improvement* of their condition with this program.

Now that you have a clear idea of your "Set Point" prior to beginning the program, let's now continue on to Chapter 24 and learn about the best way to get through those tough First Three Days.

CHAPTER REVIEW

- The power of "The Headache Relief Action Plan" is based on a uniquely integrated Mind-Body-Diet approach.

- "The Headache Relief Action Plan" is based on five "structures:" 1) Gaining knowledge of headaches; 2) Having a strategy for success; 3) Creating a personal vision statement; 4) Setting long-term goals; and 5) Establishing short-term objectives.

- Understanding how and why headaches happen, especially their chronic re-occurrence, is critical to understanding how to prevent them.

- Your personal Vision Statement ensures you define what you want to accomplish and who you wish to become.

- Goal-setting aligns your mind and body with your vision and the outcomes you desire.

- Long-term goals and short-term expectations create the foundation to keep focus and move forward in positive and productive ways.

- Metrics are essential to overcome and prevent headaches, objectively quantifying certain parts of the program, and subjectively qualifying your feelings through the journey.

CHAPTER 24

GETTING STARTED: THE FIRST THREE DAYS

The first three days of anything that requires changes are the hardest. This seems especially so when it comes to matters of health and wellness. The first three days of a new diet are a struggle, almost impossible it seems. The first three days of a new fitness program can seem unbearably painful and difficult. The first three sessions of a therapy (physical or psychological) seems to meet with the most resistance. But this doesn't have to be the case, and with an easier first three days, the chances of success are greatly improved.

One of the main reasons people claim they have started and stopped diet plans and workout routines is because they could not "get into" the program fully because the first three days were overwhelming. I have also crashed and burned within the first three days of my own health goals over the years, but was lucky to find a solution to this problem.

The problem is that most Americans want to have their cake and eat it too. In other words, they want to engage in alternative therapies like specific diets, herbal therapies, meditation, yoga sessions, mind-body modalities, and various emotional therapies; but they want the solution to be powerful and immediate (like symptomatic pain relief from analgesics). Natural solutions take longer to help the body and thus by their nature are neither toxic nor harmful in the process. More importantly, natural wellness solutions often require the person who is not well to take control and self-administer their "therapy." This is difficult for even the most sincere and holistic-minded person to do, as we have been raised to expect immediate results. Yet, fast results are not always the healthiest or longest lasting.

The solution I use with great success is to preempt those first three days with four "pre-days." That is, I start to change my thoughts about what I will begin to do, and then begin making changes to my habits and routines in small steps leading up to the first of the three days. Jumping into cold water head first can be shocking and unbearable, causing you to jump right out. However, dipping one toe in and then another and then a leg into the water, a little at a time, to prepare yourself physically, mentally, and emotionally for the inevitable jump, makes the process much easier to handle and helps make those first three days a delight to manage. Here are some things I do during the four days leading up to day one of the "first three days" of my health changing activity.

THINK FROM THE END

Before beginning a new wellness activity, I spend some time thinking about the desired result and my reasons for wanting it. Whatever the reason, I consider it, meditate on it, and think of all the wonderful things that will result from engaging in it. This gives me the emotional and mental "adjustment" towards the need and desire of what I am about to do so when the program gets tough (and they all do at times), I won't quit. Being certain of why you want something, and having a burning desire to achieve it, makes success that much easier.

GET THE SUPPORT OF OTHERS

One of the most common reasons people fall off their wellness programs is lack of support. Not only do humans tend to need to be accountable to someone, they also need to be part of a group. But often their social network is not on the same wellness path and can derail efforts by not respecting your changing needs and behaviors. I always tell my loved ones and co-workers before I begin a new program, and also ask them to ask me about my daily progress. Often people who need to change cannot do so on their own, but when a group of people in different places (work or home) ask them about it, they feel accountable and are more apt to do it. Additionally, if I am fasting or changing my diet, I ask for support and buy-in from family and friends to understand and respect my changes and not be upset with me for not eating what they may be preparing for a meal.

ADJUST YOUR "SET POINT"

I refer to a "set point" as your metric on a topic. For instance, six hours of sleep per night, three meals a day, 25 crunches; anything that can be measured by repetitions, hours, days, weight or otherwise. For many people beginning a diet, their food set point can be measured in terms of meals per day, servings per meal, number of items or counts of calories, carbs or fats per meal, etc.

The concept here is to know where you need to be during the first three days of a new diet (for example). Then mitigate that stress and diet change jump-off point, but ease into it four days prior to the start. The same goes for stretching, exercise, meditation, and anything else. Begin readjusting your less-healthy "set point" so the drastic change required of the new activity will not need as strong a shift and will be easier on the mind and body to handle and stick with it.

CHANGE YOUR ENVIRONMENT

Another difficult piece that pulls many away from ultimate success is your living environment. If you are starting a diet, but have juices with high fructose corn syrup in the fridge, frozen pizza in the freezer, white bread on the counters, and coffee calling your name, these items need to be removed. "Out of sight, out of mind" is a great saying that addresses the issue of psychological triggers. We often move on habit without thinking. Removing the unhealthy food from sight (or throwing it in the trash), putting the coffee pot into the closet, covering the TV (to help stay off the couch when we need to be out walking), and so on, helps reduce the subconscious triggers that arise from seeing things that are counterproductive to a new endeavor. If altering sleep is your issue, take the television and books out of your room prior to beginning a new sleep program. If engaging in therapies like EFT, EMDR or The Sedona Method for changing past memories and emotional triggers, remove items and pictures and music from your surroundings that may trigger and set you back in your success and interfere with moving past the first three days and into the easier fourth day and beyond.

BE SPECIFIC ON WHAT THE FIRST THREE DAYS ENTAIL

One of the best things you can do to support your ability to manage and get through those first three days is knowing exactly what you need to do and what you need to support those actions. For a cleanse or diet, it means having all the food, juice or supplements you'll need to sail through those first three days and onward from the first minute of day one. Having the food and items at your fingertips from "go" makes the start and journey through the first days easier. Without having to think, shop, and scrounge to do what's required, the mental strain is lifted, the anxiety of not knowing what to do is eased, and only the emotional and physiological aspects are left to contend with. But, if you have been shifting the emotional set-point and other areas for the four days prior, as suggested, then those issues will be less of a strain and those first three days will be much easier, if not "painless."

The four pre-days leading up to the first three days of a new wellness program are key to helping enhance the process, make the transition on your mind, emotions and body easier, and help you adjust little-by-little so the deep-end dive many do on day one will not drown them and their sincere efforts. With a four-day pre-set, the first three days can actually be a delight, and day one becomes day five.

CHAPTER REVIEW

- The first three days will be the hardest. Know the program gets easier with each passing day, week, and month.

- Failures in diets, workouts, and other challenging programs happen when those first three days are too difficult or "unbearable."

- You can succeed in the first three days of "The Headache Relief Action Plan," and it will not be as hard as most think.

- Start changing your thoughts, make changes to habits and routines in small steps, and you'll be ready to succeed before you even start your first day.

- Key strategies to prepare yourself for success involve thinking with the end goal in mind, getting support, adjusting your "set point," changing your environment, and specifying what the first three days will entail.

- You can do it!

CHAPTER 25

STEP-BY-STEP: THE 30-DAY HEADACHE RELIEF ACTION PLAN

Now it is time to put into harmonious action the hundreds of pieces of information presented in this book into a wellness lifestyle that supports relief from headaches and migraines. Below are charts outlining the seven major categories discussed in this book, and the solutions associated with each.

Implementing solutions from each of these categories forms the essence of "The Headache Relief Action Plan." The charts give you guidance into selecting the best options within each category. You must, however, review the individual chapters to find the specific details of each solution and consider which resonate best with you.

1 – DIETARY SOLUTIONS

1) Eat only pH neutral, alkalizing, and anti-inflammatory foods.

2) Drink enough pure water daily so your urine stream is clear.

3) Drink up to four cups of green tea daily, but no coffee or black tea.

4) Cook with a variety of thermogenic spices.

5) Refer to Chapters 1, 5, and 9 for details.

2 – SUPPLEMENTATION SOLUTIONS

1) Take a daily supplement to help reduce pain and inflammation.

2) Take a daily supplement to helps support blood and nerve health.

3) Select a supplement that contains enzymes and minerals.

4) Drink plenty of herbal teas that contain the herbs mentioned in Chapter 10.

5) Refer to Chapter 10 for details.

3 – ANCIENT EXERCISE SOLUTIONS

1) Get up, get moving, and remain active.

2) Start with walking and work your way up slowly.

3) Do as much as you can without triggering headache pain.

4) Begin gently and slowly, increase in time and rigor.

5) Start with mindful walking and Qigong standing.

6) If you can do more, add yoga and tai chi.

7) Refer to Chapter 16 for details.

4 – STRETCHING & BODYWORK SOLUTIONS

1) Stretching the neck and shoulders several times daily is a great release.
2) Bodywork and stretching help to relieve spasm and increase range of motion.
3) Check local listings for bodywork practitioners in your area.
4) Experience many different methods of bodywork to find what works best for you.
5) Don't be afraid of a little discomfort for long-term gain!
6) Refer to Chapter 15 for details.

5 – ENERGY MEDICINE SOLUTIONS

1) The body is electric energy vibrating at specific frequencies.
2) Pain, illness, and disease are low human vibrations.
3) Raise your frequency to vibrate in a healthy, pain-free state.
4) Experience many methods of raising vibrations to find the best one for you.
5) Some methods apply touch while other do not; be open minded.
6) Refer to Chapter 17 for details.

6 – STRESS, SLEEP, AND EMOTIONAL SOLUTIONS

1) The mind-body connection is very real.
2) Change your sleeping environment to get a restful night's sleep.

3) Use the insomnia techniques to help you get to sleep.

4) Use the recommended "10 stress busters" daily, as often as needed.

5) Practice the relaxation response or mindful meditation to release stress.

6) Use methods like EFT, EMDR and others to release repressed emotions.

7) Refer to Chapters 11, 12, 13, and 14 for details.

IMPORTANT NOTES

It is important that you include at least one thing from each of the six steps listed above in your daily life.

I highly recommend revamping your diet completely, and jumping right in with allocated times for "ancient exercises," stress reduction techniques, practitioner based bodywork, and energy medicine therapies.

I highly recommend setting appointments and times before day 1, as discussed in Chapter 21, and having several different supplements and intervention printouts on hand.

Ideally, all of the above-listed six steps should be approached at the same time. Yes, you can ease into them one per week or so, but the results will take longer. And please don't forget that assessing each area with metrics (Chapter 23), and updating those metrics weekly for the first 30 days is very important.

You might have noticed that the subtitle of the book is "30-Days to Lasting Relief from Headaches and Migraines" and yet the Headache Metrics Chart has spaces for 90 days. The program for change and successful relief of symptoms takes 30 days. It takes about 30 days for most people to grasp all that needs to be done

Step-by-Step: The 30-Day Headache Relief Action Plan

and implement and fold it into their daily lives. However, because everyone is different and requires a slightly different approach (e.g., different dietary changes, respond to different therapies, react better to different supplements and topical pain creams), adjustments need to be made for optimal outcomes. So it is a 30-day relief program that uses metrics to adjust the plan trajectory to garner best program synergy by the third month (90 days).

In other words, the first 30 days sets the tone, adjusts the attitude, reduces the stress, changes the diet, and welcomes new exercises and treatment modalities. Reduction in pain and inflammation and increased range of motion will be felt. But with a little patience and with some mindful attention to what is working best for you, you can adjust the "solutions" specifically for stronger results. You will know the results because of the metrics. By the third month you should be well on your way to once again finding homeostasis, a healthy and balanced body and life that is full of joy.

"The Headache Relief Action Plan" works because it addresses the five essential components outlined in my "Personal Message" at the start of the book. These contain the elements for positive outcomes. It is my hope that the information in the book has accomplished the following:

- ✓ Educated you about the real causes and solutions of arthritis
- ✓ Reduced the current level of symptoms you are experiencing
- ✓ Halts or significantly reduces the worsening of your condition
- ✓ Prevents symptoms from flaring to improve your quality of life

- ✓ Regenerates healthy tissue to reverse the damage done

All you have to do to see positive results is…

- ✓ Take personal responsibility for your personal arthritic condition.
- ✓ Keep educating yourself by reading and re-reading this book and online articles.
- ✓ Adjust your diet to one that is anti-inflammatory and immune building.
- ✓ Take supplements and apply topical products as needed to support symptomatic change.
- ✓ Practice ancient exercises and receive bodywork to help move blood and heal tissue.
- ✓ Receive some energy medicinal help to open energy pathways and energize.
- ✓ Practice stress relief methods and adopt better sleeping habits.
- ✓ Resolve the emotional issues that negatively impact your life.

MOST IMPORTANT: KNOW YOUR TRIGGERS

The headache triggers I discussed in Part Two include mild oxygen deprivation, chronic dehydration, toxic diet, improper exercise and rest, tight muscles, poor posture, stress, and emotions. The secret to understanding these triggers is recognizing how they cause you problems in combination with each other.

Yes, it is true that all of the above are known headache triggers. It is also true that not all of them cause headaches for you. That should be good news. But what you need to work out for yourself is which of these triggers set off your headaches and in what combination. This takes a bit of effort and commitment on your part, but is well worth it in the end. Trust me. Read on to discover how you can identify your headache triggers..

Consider each of the trigger categories, and choose one to work on for a week. If you start with oxygen deprivation, then make that your focus for each hour of each day for a week. Make sure your home and office are well-ventilated. Make a point of stopping what you are doing every hour to inhale deeply and take full breaths. Do your best to sleep in a way that does not disrupt the flow of air into your nose. See how you feel and make notes.

Then, next week, continue your oxygen program on autopilot. It should be in a self-sustaining groove so you can now focus for an entire week on hydration. This includes drinking two glasses of room temperature water each morning. You should also avoid diuretic beverages for the week (coffee, tea, soda, alcohol and beer). Drink enough water throughout the day so your urine is clear in color every time you relieve yourself. Be sure to hydrate after exercise. Again, see how you feel, take notes and then move on to changing your diet and so on.

KNOW YOUR NUMBER

After you have spent six weeks on these kinds of measures (one week for each trigger component), you should feel amazing. However, I know that many headache sufferers are in great pain and on the verge of giving up hope. Even if you have not done the above mini-program, there is still hope – if you can count.

Not all known headache triggers cause headaches in every person who gets headaches. Coffee may cause an instant headache in one person while another can drink an entire pot with no pain. This leads many to dismiss the list of triggers and think that their headaches are somehow special and unique. Again, they are not.

The secret to applying the trigger prevention method is to know your number. That is, every headache sufferer has a certain number of triggers his or her body can handle or process in a given day without problem. However, once that number is passed, you may be hit with a headache. For me, that crucial number is three.

On any given day, my body can safely handle three triggers. If I stay within that number, I will not get a headache. However, if I encounter four or more triggers, I am in pain almost immediately.

For example, if I decide to start my day with coffee and add sugar and milk (three of my triggers), I need to be extra mindful of the rest of my daily activities and choices. If I wake up with clogged sinuses (a trigger) and want coffee, then I drink it black. This allows me to remain headache-free, even if I incur one more trigger during the day. If the day is stressful, which I may not have control over, that's my third trigger. If I allow a fourth, I am out for the count with head pain.

Your number, then, is a threshold not to be passed. Everyone has a different number, but most are fewer than five. If you are able to stay within your daily number, you can prevent your headaches and thus be "cured" of them. When you surpass your number and get a headache, at least you'll know the cause and not be fooled into believing that you have no control over them or that they are unbeatable.

BENEFICIAL CORRECTIONS

Take a shot at eliminating headache triggers and find your number. If you can spend six weeks correcting these triggers, then you will be in a better place for change. If you can't do that kind of six-week program, then keep a diary of your choices, activities, and foods each day, numbering them and associating those numbers with headache intensity. That enables you to learn how to prevent them.

Most headaches are preventable because we bring them on ourselves. Stop hurting yourself, be kinder to yourself, and know your number. Here's to your headache-free life!

I know this seems like a lot, but it really isn't. Actually, it's simply a refocus of your life. More simply put, it is about adopting a well-based lifestyle that is easy to follow once you are in the groove of it, so to speak.

I wish you the best of luck and much success on your journey to a better, more joyous and pain-free life!

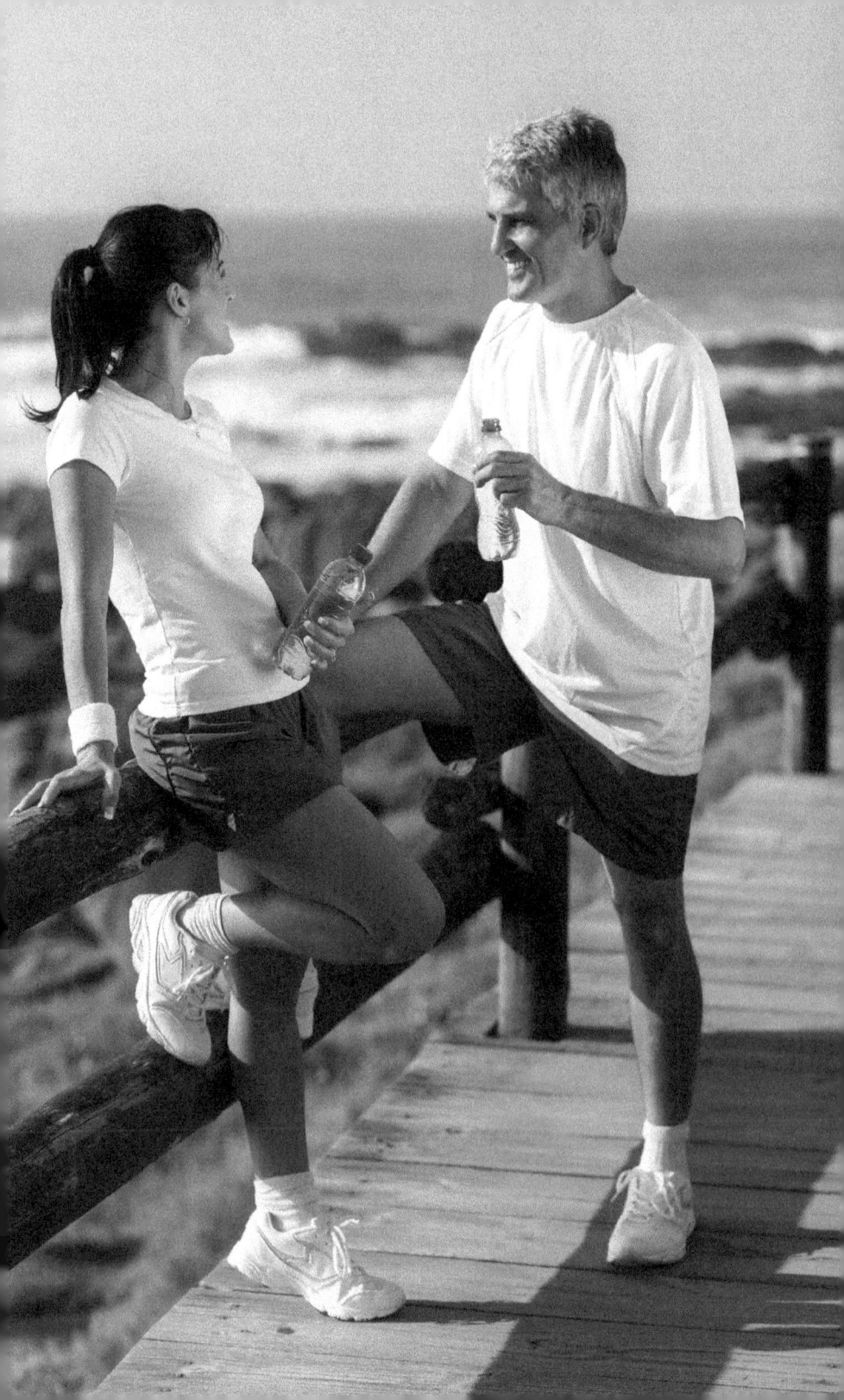

AFTERWORD

Health is not merely the absence of disease. A bevy of other lifestyle factors — including physical health, happiness, fitness, thoughts, relationships and so much more — come together to contribute to a symbiotic relationship in which your health is greatly affected by your "quality of life" — and vice versa.

This past September, the American Heart Associating (AHA) published a scientific statement that is of profound importance: "A healthy lifestyle is fundamental to the prevention and treatment of cardiovascular disease and other non-communicable diseases. Investments in primary prevention, including modification of health risk behaviors, could result in a 4-fold improvement in health outcomes compared with secondary prevention based on pharmacological treatment."

This is so important because it is rare that a science-based medical group pushes for a do-it-yourself, natural, behavior-based prevention and treatment model. Usually, their model of "wellness" is based on "correcting illness" after the fact.

For better or worse, there are so many choices we make each day that affect our quality of life and impact our health. Interestingly, they all are rooted in behaviors, and include sleeping patterns, eating patterns, food choices, stress reduction, posture, interpersonal interactions, frequency of intimacy, frequency of exercise, hydration, creative outlets, worry, anxiety, and so many more.

We have come to a point in our society and lives where it is evident that we cannot expect others to do for us what we must do for ourselves. While advances in surgical procedures are astounding, and, while we are living longer than at any other time in history, we are also suffering greatly along the way. It should be evident by now that where non-biologically induced headaches are concerned, we have personal control over most of the causes (triggers) of our chronic suffering. With some thought, planning, and changes, we can control our condition, and it is only we who can rid the headaches from our own lives. In other words, we are both the cause and cure, and it is our choice which one choose to be.

If you choose to be your own best friend and not your most feared foe, you must embrace the integrated mind-body-diet "Headache Relief Action Plan" presented in this book. And the success of this approach to curing headaches is absolutely rooted in the positive modification of your lifestyle and worldview. Without changing how you perceive the world around you, you will never live a headache-free life. The pain will keep recurring, over and over, and the more medicine you take to deaden the pain, the more you will exacerbate the condition and the worse and more damaging it will become.

I urge you to read this book several times over the next few weeks. Come to understand why and how the program works so you will believe in it because you understanding it and it makes sense to you. If you can believe in the program's abilities and you can believe in your own willingness and stamina to follow it through, it will become habitual and your lifestyle will change as necessary without painful effort. I want you to follow this program because I traveled the world in search of a cure and developed one based on the methods and research of physicians and healers and my own personal experience as a severe headache sufferer for over 30 dreadful years. I want you to be pain free, too, and I know it will happen if you dedicate the necessary time, energy and love to yourself.

I wish you much success and happiness for the rest of your healthy and headache-free life.

REFERENCES

Introduction

1. WHO. "Headache Disorders." http://www.who.int/mediacentre/factsheets/fs277/en/

Chapter 1

1. Mukamal, KJ, Wellenius GA, et al. (2009). "Weather and air pollution as triggers of severe headaches." *Neurology* vol. 72, no. 10 922-927. http://www.neurology.org/content/72/10/922

2. Robert T. (2016). "Impact of Air Pollution on Migraines and Headaches." Health Central. http://www.healthcentral.com/migraine/triggers-530998-5.html

Chapter 2

1. National Headache Foundation "Fact Sheet." http://www.health-exchange.net/pdfdb/headfactEng.pdf

2. National Association of Neurological Disorders and Stroke. "Migraine Information Page." https://www.ninds.nih.gov/Disorders/All-Disorders/Migraine-Information-Page

Chapter 3

1. *New England Journal of Medicine.* http://www.nejm.org/

2. Centers for Disease Control and Prevention. "Injury Prevention & Control: Opioid Overdose." https://www.cdc.gov/drugoverdose/data/fentanyl.html

3. *Journal of Headache and Pain.* "Risk of medication overuse headache across classes of treatments for acute migraine." http://thejournalofheadacheandpain.springeropen.com/articles/10.1186/s10194-016-0696-8

Chapter 4

1. Migraine Research Foundation. "Migraine is an extraordinarily prevalent neurological disease, affecting 38 million men, women and children in the U.S. and 1 billion worldwide." https://migraineresearchfoundation.org/about-migraine/migraine-facts/

2. Health Central. "Migraine and Headache Burden: New WHO Report." http://www.healthcentral.com/migraine/support-580267-5.html

3. World Health Organizations. "Atlas of Headache Disorders and Resources in the World 2011." http://www.who.int/mental_health/management/atlas_headache_disorders/en/

Chapter 9

1. pH Spectrum Graphic - mindbodygreen.com http://www.mindbodygreen.com/0-5165/Alkaline-Acidic-Foods-Chart-The-pH-Spectrum.html

2. Batmanghelidj, F. (1996). *Your Body's Many Cries for Water.* Falls Church, VA: Global Health Solutions.

3. Milne, R., More, B. et al. (1997). *Definitive Guide to Headaches.* Tiburon, CA: Future Medicine Publishing

4. United States Environmental Protection Agency. "How Safe is My Drinking Water?" www.epa.gov/safewater/wrot/howsafe.html

5. Janovy, CJ. (2013). "Chemical commonly found in plastics makes migraines worse, researchers show." KU Medical Center News. http://www.kumc.edu/news-listing-page/researchers-show-connection-between-bisphenol-a-and-migraine.html

Chapter 10

1. Estemalik E, Tepper S (2013). "Preventive treatment in migraine and the new US guidelines." *Journal of Neuropsychiatric Disease and Treatment.* https://www.ncbi.nlm.nih.gov/pmc/articles/PMC3663475/

2. Sewell RA. (2008). "Response of Cluster Headache to Kudzu." *Headache: Journal of Head and Face Pain.* http://onlinelibrary.wiley.com/doi/10.1111/j.1526-4610.2008.01268.x/full

3. National Sleep Foundation. "Melatonin and Sleep." https://sleepfoundation.org/sleep-topics/melatonin-and-sleep

4. Gonçalves AL, Ferreira AM, Ribeiro RT, et al. (2016). "Randomised clinical trial comparing melatonin 3 mg, amitriptyline 25 mg and placebo for migraine prevention." *Journal of Neurology, Neurosurgery & Psychology.* http://jnnp.bmj.com/content/early/2016/05/10/jnnp-2016-313458.abstract

Chapter 11

1. Freeman, L.W. & Lawlis, G.F. (2001). *Mosby's Complementary and Alternative Medicine: A Research-based Approach.* St. Louis, MO: Mosby.

2. Benson H. (1976). *The Relaxation Response.* Harper Torch.

3. Wells RE, Burch R, Paulsen RH, et al. (2014). "Meditation for migraines: a pilot randomized controlled trial." *Headache*, 54 (9): 1484-95.

4. Azam MA, Katz J, Mohabir V, Ritvo R. (2016). "Individuals with tension and migraine headaches exhibit increased heart rate variability during post-stress mindfulness meditation practice but a decrease during a post-stress control condition - A randomized, controlled experiment." *International Journal of Psychophysiology*. https://www.ncbi.nlm.nih.gov/pubmed/27769879

Chapter 12

1. Reed, Daniel. (1998). *Chi-Kung: Harnessing the Power of the Universe*. Great Britain: Simon and Schuster.

2. Stagliano. (1991). *The D.O.* p. 86.

3. Milne, R., More, B. et al. (1997). *Definitive Guide to Headaches*. Tiburon, CA: Future Medicine Publishing

Chapter 13

1. Milne, R., More, B. et al. (1997). *Definitive Guide to Headaches*. Tiburon, CA: Future Medicine Publishing

2. Baran B, Pace-Schott F, Ericson C, et al. (2012). "Processing of Emotional Reactivity and Emotional Memory over Sleep." *Journal of Neuroscience, 32 (3)*.

Chapter 14

1. Tolle E. "The Pain Body." http://communicate.eckharttolle.com/news/2014/08/13/when-the-pain-body-awakens/

2. Driessen E, Hollon SD, Bockting CLH, et al. (2015). "Does Publication Bias Inflate the Apparent Efficacy of Psychological Treatment for Major Depressive Disorder? A Systematic Review and Meta-Analysis of US National Institutes of Health-Funded Trials." *PLOS One*. http://journals.plos.org/plosone/article?id=10.1371/journal.pone.0137864

3. Marino K. (2012). *Breaking Free From Critical Addiction: Our #1 Social Disease*. Balbo Press.

4. Shapiro F. (2012). *Getting Past Your Past: Take Control of Your Life with Self-Help Techniques from EMDR Therapy*. Rodale.

5. Sarno J. (2010). *Healing Back Pain*. Grand Central.

Chapter 16

1. *Traditional Chinese Therapeutic Exercises – Standing Pole,* by Wang Xuanjei and J.P.C. Moffett

2. Brown NP. (2010). "Easing Ills through Tai Chi." *Harvard Magazine*. http://harvardmagazine.com/2010/01/researchers-study-tai-chi-benefits

Chapter 17

1. "Acupuncture More Effective than Medication for Headache Relief." Duke Medicine News and Communications. http://www.balancingpointacupuncture.com/wordpress/wp-content/uploads/2012/02/AcupunctureMoreEffectivethanMedicationforHeadacheRelief.pdf?99e69a

2. "Expressions of Concern from Scientists, Physicians, Health Policy Experts & Others." Electromagnetic Health. http://electromagnetichealth.org/quotes-from-experts/

3. Piquet M, Balestra C, et al. (2010). "Supraorbital transcutaneous neurostimulation has sedative effects in healthy subjects." *BMC Neurology.* http://bmcneurol.biomedcentral.com/articles/10.1186/1471-2377-11-135

4. Magis D, Sava S, et al. (2013). "Safety and patients' satisfaction of transcutaneous Supraorbital NeuroStimulation (tSNS) with the Cefaly® device in headache treatment: a survey of 2,313 headache sufferers in the general population." *Journal of Headache and Pain.* https://thejournalofheadacheandpain.springeropen.com/articles/10.1186/1129-2377-14-95

5. FDA News Release. (2013). "FDA Allows Marketing of First Device to Relieve Migraine Headache Pain." http://www.fda.gov/NewsEvents/Newsroom/PressAnnouncements/ucm378608.htm

Chapter 18

1. Mandato K and Lipton RB. March 1, 2015, Society of Interventional Radiology Meeting, Atlanta, GA.

2. https://hms.harvard.edu/news/green-light-migraine-relief

3. Noseda R, Bernstein CA, et al. (2016). "Migraine Photophobia Originating in Cone-driven Retinal Pathways." *Brain: A Journal of Neurology.* http://brain.oxfordjournals.org/content/early/2016/05/16/brain.aww119

4. Borgelt LM, Ferason KL, et al. (2013). "The Pharmacologic and Clinical Effects of Medical Cannabis." *Pharmacotherapy*. http://onlinelibrary.wiley.com/doi/10.1002/phar.1187/abstract

5. "Where Is Marijuana Legal in the United States? List of Recreational and Medicinal States." https://mic.com/articles/126303/where-is-marijuana-legal-in-the-united-states-list-of-recreational-and-medicinal-states#.2wI8T1P4o

Afterword

1. "Quality of Life as Prognostic Measure: Analysis suggests association between QoL and outcomes." MedPage Today. http://www.medpagetoday.com/mastery-of-medicine/cardiology-mastery-in-chf/61203?xid=nl_mpt_DHE_2016-11-03&eun=g713345d0r&pos=1

DR. MARK WILEY, SELF-DIRECTED WELLNESS EXPERT

Dr. Mark V. Wiley PhD, OMD is an internationally renowned mind-body health advocate, author, and publisher. He has spent decades traveling extensively throughout the United States, Europe and Asia to research, experience, learn and master the world's alternative and natural healing practices; from the oldest to the most modern.

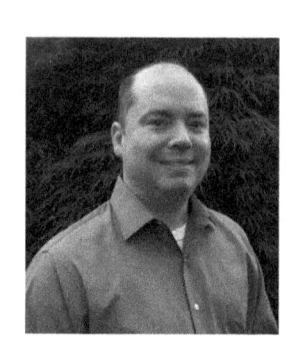

Dr. Mark's interest in alternative health practices was not just a mere curiosity; he was looking for long-lasting relief from the debilitating migraines and chronic pain that plagued him from childhood. He received treatments from medical doctors, psychologists, chiropractors, physical therapists, hypnotists, acupuncturists, herbalists, bone-setters, Qigong masters, yoga masters, traditional Chinese doctors, faith healers and tribal shamans. None of them, individually, were able to offer him lasting relief from his daily torment. So he took it upon himself to learn their methods, in the process earning a Master's in Health Care Management and Doctorate's in both Alternative Medicine and Oriental Medicine.

This experience and education led Dr. Mark to develop methods of uncovering root causes, relieving and then preventing – not just "treating" – physical ailments, such as migraines, back pain and arthritis, as well as conditions like hypertension, obesity, fatigue and other health concerns. His integrated mind-body approach synthesizes decades of research and personal experience, focusing on balancing the body – returning it to homeostasis – thereby providing recovery, balance, and prevention of adverse health conditions. This happens because the environment that allows the condition or disease to exist is no longer present. This is the treatment Dr. Mark used to bring his own migraines and chronic pain under control, and this is the method he promotes in his work to help others in need.

In addition to writing and publishing about health and wellness, Dr. Mark has interviewed for print and radio in the U.S., U.K. and Asia, lecturing at various universities, and teaching at holistic healing centers. He has written 15 books and more than 700 articles.

Today he serves on the health advisory boards of several wellness centers and associations while focusing his attention on helping people achieve healthy and balanced lives through his work with The Healthy Back Institute, Easy Health Options® and his company, Tambuli Media.

Sign up to receive Dr. Wiley's FREE weekly Email Newsletter for great wellness articles and discount codes for other great health and wellness books.

https://tambulimedia.activehosted.com/f/11

"EXCELLENCE IN MIND/BODY PUBLISHING"

TAMBULI MEDIA

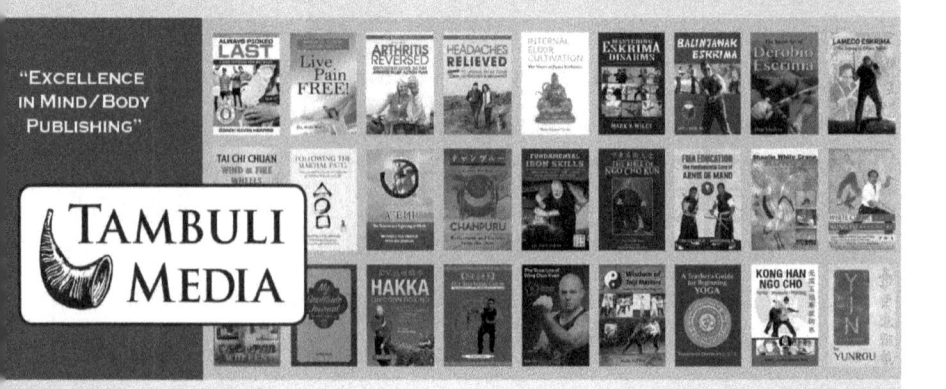

Welcome to **Tambuli Media**, publisher of quality books and digital media on lifestyle, health, fitness, and traditional martial arts.

Our Vision is to see mind-body practices once again playing an integral role in the lives of people who pursue a journey of personal development to improve their lives and inspire others.

Our Mission is to partner with the highest caliber subject-matter experts to bring you quality content that is in-depth, professional, actionable and comprehensive in nature. We welcome you to join our Tambuli Family and to spend time on our site reading articles, watching videos, downloading content, and ordering products. Join one or more of our Email Lists to stay in touch and receive "Members Only" content, invitations to private webinars, and discount codes on new releases and bundled merchandise.

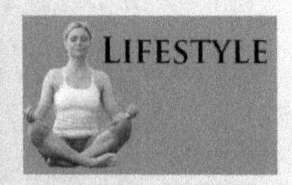

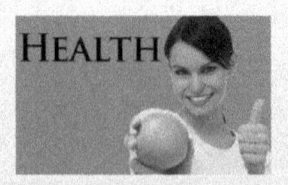

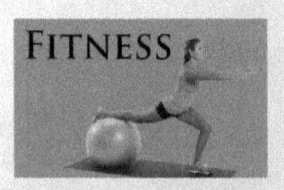

LIFESTYLE   HEALTH   FITNESS

FILIPINO MARTIAL ARTS   CHINESE MARTIAL ARTS   JAPANESE OKINAWAN MARTIAL ARTS

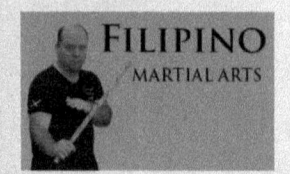

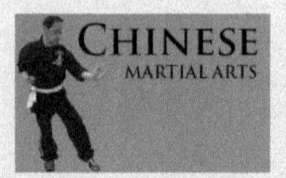

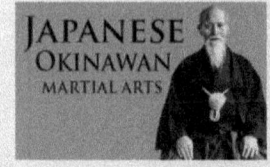

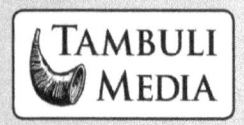

TAMBULI MEDIA
www.tambulimedia.com